# Janet Evans' Total Swimming

Janet Evans

Human Kinetics

**Library of Congress Cataloging-in-Publication Data**

Evans, Janet, 1971-
  Janet Evans' total swimming / Janet Evans.
    p. cm.
  Includes bibliographical references and index.
  ISBN-13: 978-0-7360-6848-2 (soft cover)
  ISBN-10: 0-7360-6848-1 (soft cover)
  1. Swimming--Training. 2. Evans, Janet, 1971-
3. Swimming--Anecdotes. I. Title.
  GV837.7.E83 2007
  797.2'1--dc22                    2007008514

ISBN-10: 0-7360-6848-1
ISBN-13: 978-0-7360-6848-2

The Web addresses cited in this text were current as of February, 2007, unless otherwise noted.

**Acquisitions Editor:** Jana Hunter; **Developmental Editor:** Amanda Eastin; **Assistant Editor:** Christine Horger; **Copyeditor:** John Wentworth; **Proofreader:** Anne Rogers; **Indexer:** Craig Brown; **Graphic Designer:** Nancy Rasmus; **Graphic Artist:** Kim McFarland; **Cover Designer:** Keith Blomberg; **Photographer (cover):** John Strand; **Photographer (interior):** John Strand, unless otherwise noted; **Photos:** Jason Allen; **Printer:** United Graphics

We thank the Marguerite Aquatic Center in Mission Viejo, California, for assistance in providing the location for the photo shoot for this book.

Human Kinetics books are available at special discounts for bulk purchase. Special editions or book excerpts can also be created to specification. For details, contact the Special Sales Manager at Human Kinetics.

Printed in the United States of America     10  9  8  7  6  5  4  3  2  1

**Human Kinetics**
Web site: www.HumanKinetics.com

*United States:* Human Kinetics
P.O. Box 5076
Champaign, IL 61825-5076
800-747-4457
e-mail: humank@hkusa.com

*Canada:* Human Kinetics
475 Devonshire Road Unit 100
Windsor, ON N8Y 2L5
800-465-7301 (in Canada only)
e-mail: orders@hkcanada.com

*Europe:* Human Kinetics
107 Bradford Road
Stanningley
Leeds LS28 6AT, United Kingdom
+44 (0) 113 255 5665
e-mail: hk@hkeurope.com

*Australia:* Human Kinetics
57A Price Avenue
Lower Mitcham, South Australia 5062
08 8372 0999
e-mail: liaw@hkaustralia.com

*New Zealand:* Human Kinetics
Division of Sports Distributors NZ Ltd.
P.O. Box 300 226 Albany
North Shore City
Auckland
0064 9 448 1207
e-mail: info@humankinetics.co.nz

*For Billy, the best training partner I could ask for.*

# contents

# acknowledgments

In acknowledging those who have been my inspiration for writing this book, I find that many of them have been instrumental in my athletic career as well. First and foremost, I want to thank my parents, Barbara and Paul, who took me to swim lessons when I was 18 months old and spent the next 24 years supporting my dreams. Then there are my coaches. After all, they are the ones who taught me the majority of the lessons in this book. To Mrs. White—my first swim teacher—thank you for teaching me all four strokes before my third birthday. To my stroke coach, Mr. John Virgo, thank you for teaching me that a positive attitude is imperative to success. To Bud McAllister, Don Wagner, and Tom Milich, thank you for giving me the confidence to win gold medals and break world records while I was in high school. And to Mark Schubert, thank you for your patience and support as I trained for my final two Olympic Games.

Outside of the pool, there are others I need to thank, especially Jana Hunter, who envisioned this book, and my agent Evan Morgenstein, who encouraged me to write it and gave me confidence that it could be done. I thank my daughter Sydney Grace, who swam with me stroke for stroke for the entire nine months of my pregnancy. And, finally, this book would not be possible without my husband, Billy Willson, who began swimming when we met and is now one of the most passionate masters swimmers I know. Because of him, I found myself back in the pool years after my retirement, enjoying the sport more than I thought possible. This book was written with him in mind.

# introduction

The benefits of swimming are numerous, significant, and undeniable. Swimming can be beneficial to people across a broad range of ages and abilities: the very young to the very old, the very slow to the very fast, those with injuries or degenerative conditions, pregnant women, beginner to serious athletes, and fitness buffs. Swimming positively affects many aspects of life, including physical, mental, and emotional well-being. It's no wonder that physicians, physical therapists, exercise physiologists, and fitness coaches alike laud swimming as one of the best ways to stay in shape.

Swimming is the ultimate all-in-one fitness package, working most muscles in the body in a variety of ways with every stroke. When strokes are performed correctly, the muscles lengthen and increase in flexibility. The significant repetition of strokes improves muscle endurance, and because water creates more resistance against the body than air does in land exercise, the muscles are strengthened and toned. Swimming also significantly enhances core strength, which is important to overall health and stability in everyday life. The hip, back, and abdominal muscles are crucial to moving through the water effectively and efficiently. Swimming builds these core muscles better than any abs video or gadget advertised on television. Finally, a properly structured swim workout provides incredible improvements to the cardiovascular system. The nature of breathing when swimming—with breath being somewhat limited in volume and frequency—promotes greater lung capacity and a consistent intake of oxygen. Both aerobic and anaerobic gains can be made in the same workout.

Compare all this to other activities, which offer benefits to only certain parts of the body or areas of fitness. Running increases cardiovascular fitness and tones the lower body. Rowing builds endurance and strength in both the upper body and lower body. Weightlifting tones or builds strength in the muscles targeted. Pilates and yoga improve core strength and flexibility. But the beauty of swimming is that it literally does all of the above in every single workout! When you're a swimmer, there's no need to choose each day whether you'll focus on your upper body or lower body, muscular strength or cardiovascular endurance, core strength or overall flexibility. Swimming also is easy on the body, as long as a proper warm-up and cool-down are incorporated into each session. The pounding the body takes during running, high-impact aerobics, basketball, tennis, and kickboxing is replaced by near weightlessness in the water. In short, consistent swimming tones the body, improves cardiovascular health, and lengthens the muscles, all without breaking down the body.

Swimming is also good for the mind and spirit. The methodical repetition of swimming combined with its nonimpact nature creates a soothing, relaxing form of exercise. A good swim can clear the mind after a tough day at work, calm the spirit with a sense of quietness to give the brain a chance to sneak up on problems with creative solutions, and give you time to catch up with elusive ideas. Swimming is a great way to be alone in a world that increasingly demands that we be available to anyone and everyone 24-7. Carrying a cell phone or pager is totally feasible on land—and reaching the point where it's almost expected—but you can't swim with a PDA strapped to your chest like a heart-rate monitor. In addition, swimming for more than 20 minutes or so signals the body to release pain-killing, euphoria-producing endorphins that promote a keen sense of well-being. Regular swim workouts help on an emotional level, too. The discipline it takes to commit to swimming and to push yourself through tough workouts improves self-esteem, instills confidence that other challenges or hurdles can be overcome, and inspires dedication to taking care of yourself in all facets of life. All of this culminates into feeling really good about yourself, inside and out.

Besides the physical and mental benefits provided, swimming has many practical advantages over other forms of exercise. As long as lifeguards are present, swimming is extremely safe. Swimmers don't risk getting hit by a car or chased by a dog; they never have to choose between finishing a workout and being alone in a dark or dangerous area; and they don't have to wonder when the equipment was last sanitized. Also, workouts can be completed with equal ease alone, with a partner, or with a group of swimmers. Environmental conditions are relatively consistent regardless of time of day or year, so the amount of equipment, preparation, or planning changes very little. Swimming for fitness is also relatively inexpensive. The amount of gear can be quite minimal, and the most useful gear is inexpensive and durable. There is no fancy equipment or machine to maintain. The cost of using a pool is comparable to that of joining a gym or health club, and often the facility offers additional perks such as weight equipment or group classes that come standard with facilities that have a pool.

I believe the benefits of swimming are enough to make everyone want to rush out to buy a suit and appropriate gear and to begin swimming every day of the week! Physically, you'd become as fit as ever; mentally, you'd slow the effects of aging and begin solving problems in a single workout; and emotionally, you'd be on a constant swimmer's high. But, as we all know, it never works out quite like that. Life happens, and even the most dedicated swimmers will encounter difficulties in keeping to their routine. Some people might struggle to find the perfect facility that has the perfect lap swim schedule. Others might cringe at the idea of getting wet in the middle of the day, of putting on a still-damp swimsuit from the previous day's workout, or of wearing a swimsuit in public in the first place (although it's amazing how quickly the awkwardness of walking from the locker room to the pool in a swimsuit fades). Even after 30 years, the hardest part for me remains simply jumping in, especially when the water or air is chilly. Despite the benefits swimming offers, the excuses or interruptions that threaten our consistency of getting any form of exercise can be daunting, especially to newer swimmers.

Regular swimmers know that sticking with an established schedule allows them to experience the all-around healthiness and well-being their workouts bring. A few motivation boosters, such as working out with a partner, joining a masters swim team, and, most important, having a plan, coupled with the knowledge of the tremendous benefits of swimming, will help beginner and veteran swimmers alike get to the pool more often and work hard once they get there.

Most people would benefit from working out with at least one other like-minded person. The single most important characteristic of a great training partner—more so than comparable ability—is comparable commitment to the activity. Differences in speed can be addressed with equipment or workout design. But a lack of dependability, such as always being late or prone to cancel, is detrimental to the concept of a workout partner. Meeting another person at a specific time is usually all the impetus needed to get there when motivation otherwise wanes. But even after getting in the pool, a buddy often makes the time there more pleasurable. Completing a full workout as written is tough some days, whether physically, mentally, or emotionally. Pushing yourself to swim hard is easier when someone else is right there testing his or her limits along with you and helping to break up the workout with friendly competitions. Afterward, it's great to have that friend to chat with about the session's high and low points and to be there for encouragement during a string of difficult sessions.

A logical progression for some fitness swimmers is to join a group of swimmers. United States Masters Swimming is a national organization open to all swimmers age 18 and over. More than 500 clubs are located around the country, and each has scheduled workout sessions developed and administered by an experienced swim coach. Swimmers of virtually any level are welcome on masters teams. The most important skills to have are understanding the lingo, being able to read workouts, and being able to read a pace clock. If the coach says to swim five 500s on 7:00, you need to know what that means and how to execute it. If the coach says it's time to pull, you need to know to put on your paddles and pull buoys. (All of this is explained in the book.) Although swimming ability varies greatly among individuals on a team, each workout entails steady swimming for 45 minutes to an hour and covers about 3,000 yards (2,743 meters). Being able to relatively easily complete a workout of 1,000 to 1,500 yards (914-1,371 meters) that includes an interval set should enable you to successfully join the team. Generally the atmosphere at masters workouts is not intense or pressure packed, so individuals get out of the sessions what they put into them. Joining a team does cost money, though the fees generally are in line with the costs of joining a health club or gym. More information can be found at www.usms.org.

Whether you get your swimming in with someone or alone, the single most significant way you can help yourself improve is to have a plan. Schedule your workouts into your day rather than let the day determine when you get to the pool. Without the premeditated effort of adding your swim workouts to your calendar every week, fitting them in will be a long shot on most days and a reality on very few.

The pages of this book are filled with information on how to reap the most benefits of your time in the pool by getting prepared and having a plan. Part I covers the various types of gear and how each piece helps you improve. The technique of each stroke—freestyle, backstroke, breaststroke, and butterfly—and their turns is broken down so you can mix up your workouts and improve your overall swimming performances. The primary concepts of swim training are explained, such as setting goals and charting workouts, the makeup of a workout, and interval training. Finally, specific exercises, routines, and drills are provided to enhance your workouts.

The meat of the book is parts II and III. Part II includes 60 workouts that vary in type, intensity, distance, and time. These workouts are broken into five categories that can give new life to your lap-swimming days, your fitness, and your rate of improvement. Part III puts it all together to provide you—regardless of your swimming season or goals—with programs to help you meet those goals. Twelve programs incorporate the 60 workouts from part II and range in length from four to eight weeks and in workout frequency from three to six days a week. The natural progression of these programs enables swimmers to move smoothly from one program to the next. The final chapter describes the purpose and nature of the various training phases so that competitors can tailor a training program to prepare for a specific race or event.

Swimming is an activity many people have done virtually their entire lives. Kids look forward to days at the pool, lake, or ocean, splashing around and racing friends. When adulthood strikes, though, our uninhibited joy of playing in the water often subsides. Our minds are filled with images of swimming lap after lap in an effort to lose weight, gain fitness, or compete in a swim meet or triathlon. My goal for this book is to make swimming enjoyable for you so you can experience a combination of the childlike enthusiasm for swimming and the adultlike result of meeting your individual goals. Whether you have been lap swimming for years, swam as a kid and want to get back in the water, or have a competitive streak for masters meets or triathlons, *Janet Evans' Total Swimming* has been written with you in mind!

# part I

# The Essentials

Swimming is one of the most popular ways to stay fit, with more than 15.6 million people swimming in the United States alone. Before you read further, stop and give yourself a pat on the back for contributing to a "good" statistic. Based on the benefits and advantages of swimming over other fitness activities noted in the introduction, you can congratulate yourself on being smart, too! But regardless of whether you've been a part of the swimming population for decades, years, months, or hours, chances are you don't know everything there is to know about how to make your experience in the pool more enjoyable and effective. Part I includes the essential information you need to do just that. With instruction, anecdotes, and artwork, there's something here for everyone.

Contrary to what it may seem, showing up at the pool is not the first step in swimming. Getting equipped is. The choices these days for everything from socks to a cup of coffee are overwhelming at times, and swimmers have not been spared the deluge of options. Swimsuits come in a variety of fabrics, cuts, and colors. Equipment such as fins and paddles come in several styles, each of which slightly alters the training focus. Not only must you decide from among many choices of pieces of gear, you also must determine what gear is vital to swimming, what gear is really good to have, and what gear clearly falls into the optional category. Finally, if you're fortunate enough to have more than one pool or body of water to swim in, knowing what to look for when making that choice is key. All of these questions and more are answered in chapter 1.

Virtually anyone who decides to swim for fitness already knows how to swim the freestyle, which is without question the most common stroke for lap swimmers. But not everyone is proficient in the freestyle, and fewer still are capable of swimming each of the other three strokes—the backstroke, breaststroke, and butterfly—with confidence. Chapter 2 provides a concise, yet complete, explanation of how to swim and to perform the turns for each stroke. The descriptions, analogies, photographs, and illustrations will help almost any swimmer improve technique and performance.

Swimming lap after lap with no variation in distance or intensity is one way to improve fitness and health, but it probably won't yield the best results. Progression in the pool is more likely if you recognize the five steps of improving as a swimmer, fully grasp the inspiration that can come with diligently logging what you do in each workout, understand the various components of a standard swim workout, realize the importance of interval training and using a pace clock, learn how to measure and then alter your effort levels at different times, and know how to prevent injuries. Look to chapter 3 for explanations of all these details.

The safest and most productive swimming workouts involve more than just jumping into the pool, swimming as hard as you can for a specified amount of time or distance, and jumping out. In addition to the warm-up and cool-down discussed in chapter 3, stretching before you even get in the water will drastically decrease the chance of injury. Exercises that build strength and endurance in the core muscles will surely help your swim technique. Details of specific stretching and core-strengthening routines, along with drills incorporated into the workouts of later chapters, are presented in chapter 4.

# chapter 1

# Swim Gear and Environments

When it comes to gear required for participation, swimming is a relatively simple sport. Swimming gear is uncomplicated and inexpensive compared to the highly technical equipment some sports require, and the venue for most swimmers is pretty standard. Pools may be indoors or outdoors, and lengths may vary somewhat, but the general features are about the same from pool to pool. Still, there are things to consider when choosing equipment and a place to swim. In this chapter we'll sort through the gear that is mandatory or strongly recommended; gear that will enhance your workouts, fitness, or technique; and any other equipment and products that might improve your experience. We will also discuss the various places to swim (indoor pools, outdoor pools, and open water), the pros and cons of each, and, to help keep peace during your time at the pool, the points of etiquette of lap swimming.

## Workout Gear

As is true of participation in most sports and activities, high-quality equipment makes the experience of swimming more enjoyable. Riding a bicycle is easier and more fun when the size of the bike suits the size of the cyclist. A family trip in a vehicle large enough for everyone to have their own space is far preferable to being crammed into a pickup.

When it comes to swimming, you'll find your motivation to return to the pool will increase once you have gear that best suits your needs. This holds true whether you're a minimalist, a gear junkie, or somewhere in between. Goggles that fit and don't leak, equipment that improves your stroke and your fitness, the smell of chlorine staying at the pool instead of following you home—such factors buoy your interest in swimming and make it more likely that you'll return to the water.

To be an avid swimmer, you don't have to spend a lot of money, although some swimmers do. In fact, the number of pieces of equipment used in swimming can be as few as *one*—a swimsuit—or as many as a dozen if you add in goggles; a cap; a pull buoy; a variety of fins and paddles for different strokes and benefits; kickboards; stretch tubes; a waterproof MP3 player; hair, skin, and suit care products; and a bag to carry it all in.

## Mandatory and Strongly Recommended Gear

Other than a body of water to swim in, a swimsuit is the only gear that's truly mandatory for swimming. Virtually every community pool, YMCA, or health club requires a swimsuit rather than simply shorts and a T-shirt or sports bra. You can swim in open water in makeshift attire, but efficiency and comfort in the water are greatly enhanced by a suit. Less essential than a swimsuit but strongly recommended is a pair of goggles. Swimming properly for any length of time or with any consistency will be difficult on the eyes without goggles to protect them from the chlorine or, in open water, from salt or bacteria. For swimmers with hair long enough to get in their eyes, or for those who want to take extra care of their hair, a swim cap is beneficial. A towel and a water bottle help to dry water off the body and put water back in, respectively, and a log book helps to chart your progress as you follow the workouts and programs in this book. This section will cover in detail each of the items mentioned and offer advice for selecting and using your gear.

### Swimsuit

For people swimming regularly for exercise and fitness, the best type of material for a swimsuit is Lycra. This stretchy, resilient, and comfortable fabric is the most commonly used in swimwear. Most stores that carry swimsuits offer Lycra suits made by several different companies, including Speedo, TYR, and Nike.

For women, styles range from a very modest high cut above the chest and low cut at the thigh with wide shoulder straps, to an open back with narrow straps, to training two-pieces that provide more coverage and comfort than fashion bikinis. Such suits typically range in price from about $35 to $75 U.S. The overall fit of the suit should be quite snug because it will stretch out a bit when wet and with use. Make sure the shoulder straps don't rub the skin where the neck meets the shoulders and that they don't dig uncomfortably into the shoulders. The cut at the hips should allow for a good range of motion, but more than anything the suit should feel comfortable and appropriate. Because of the number of brands and styles of suits, finding one that fits well and that's comfortable should be a matter of diligence rather than chance. Try on different styles and cuts of suits, and mimic your swimming strokes in the dressing room to see how a suit feels in action. This doesn't guarantee the best choice but might help narrow your options.

Compared to the factors involved in selecting a women's suit, choosing a men's suit is relatively straightforward. Again, comfort is the key. Choices of suit types available for men are fewer than for women but much larger than they used to be. For many years, men had only two options for a suit: the traditional tiny briefs or the bulky, drag-inducing trunks that make for increased coverage but decreased speed. Enter jammers in the mid-1990s. Jammers have the look of biking shorts with skin-tight Lycra covering the thigh to midthigh or the knee, depending on the cut. Men's suits of this type generally run between $20 and $35 U.S. The suit should feel comfortable on your body, and you should feel comfortable wearing the suit at the pool. Figure 1.1 shows examples of swimwear for women and men.

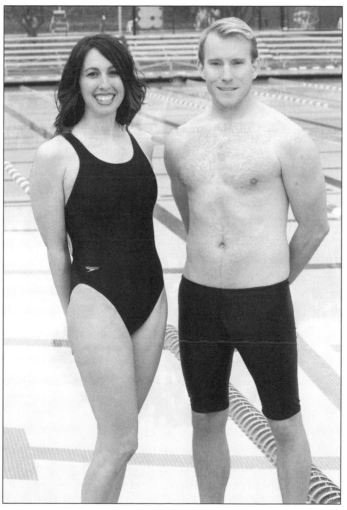

**Figure 1.1** A traditional Lycra swimsuit for women and a jammer swimsuit for men.

## Making a Suit Work

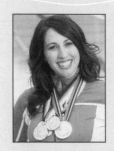

When I was 16 and swimming 12 miles a day, my training suit was a Speedo Racerback. The only problem with it—like all suits in my day—was that the straps were set relatively narrow and rubbed against my neck. Even after 2,000 yards—a relatively short distance—the suit began to irritate my neck, and by the middle portion of the workout, chafing marks would start to develop. Wanting neither to switch suits nor to have permanent scars on my neck, I tried rubbing Vaseline on my neck to ease the friction. It worked! In this day and age of option upon option, being forced to resort to such measures as Vaseline is highly unlikely, but the product is effective should you not want to part with that lucky suit.

Depending on their goals, some swimmers choose suits made of fabrics other than Lycra. At the 2000 Olympic Games in Sydney, Australia, suits made of fabric that replicates the amazing drag-resistant skin of a shark made a big splash. These suits also increase buoyancy to help maintain an optimal streamline position (discussed in the next chapter). But great performance comes at a price—in this case between $85 and $300 U.S., depending on the style of suit—and the great effort it takes to put on and take off. Elite swimmers, masters swimmers, and triathletes might find that price acceptable for two reasons. The suit could lower a swimmer's personal record by up to 7.5 percent because of reduced drag, and it could provide a small advantage over opponents without such a suit. Such a suit should be saved for the big event rather than being worn to train in. Its life will be extended significantly, and the swimmer will feel even faster when wearing it.

Speedo, a leading manufacturer of swimwear, offers another alternative to Lycra. Speedo has developed a chlorine-resistant fabric called Speedo Endurance that is reasonable in price ($30-$70 U.S.). Swimsuits wear out primarily because of the corrosive nature of chlorine. Speedo Endurance suits fade less quickly, last longer, and, because they're slightly thicker than the average Lycra suit, are more modest.

No matter what type of suit you choose, proper care will increase its lifespan and save you money. After every workout, rinse your suit out with cold water. To remove excess water, squeeze the suit rather than wring it, which breaks down the fibers more quickly. Then lay the suit flat on a towel until it's dry. After every several workouts, clean the suit by hand with a gentle soap or a suit-cleaning product. Never dry your suit in a normal clothes dryer because the heat destroys the fabric. Many pool locker rooms have special swimsuit dryers that extract water from the suit in just seconds without using heat. When cared for in this way, suits will last several months or more depending on how often you swim.

## Goggles

Goggles just miss the mandatory gear designation. Yes, people can swim without wearing goggles, and they did so for years—some with great success. In fact, 1972 Olympic sensation Mark Spitz, who won seven gold medals in Munich, didn't wear goggles while training in the mid- to late 1960s. Before the 1960s, no one wore goggles. But by the 1972 Olympics in Munich, goggles were fairly common, and the protection they provided the eyes from chlorinated pools enabled elite swimmers to train more hours daily and thus lower their times. The same holds true for nonelite swimmers. Wearing goggles indirectly improves the fitness of almost any swimmer because the increased comfort in the water decreases the chance of all but the most dedicated of cutting workouts short or skipping them altogether because of eye irritation.

As is true for swimsuits, many manufacturers make many different sizes and styles of goggles. And as with suits, it might take a bit of experimenting to find a pair that works for you. The combination of the fit of the eyepieces and head straps should prevent water from entering the lens area without being so tight to cause discomfort. Most goggles are made with foam around the eyepieces and one or two head straps to keep them in place. Many goggles can be tailored to fit. The nosepiece is often adjustable to lengthen or shorten the gap between the lenses to better fit the size and shape of different faces, and altering the length of the head straps changes the tightness of the goggles around the head. Head straps should fit around the midway point of the back of the head or slightly higher for best results. For the competitive swimmer who is looking for every advantage possible, Swedish goggles (or imitations thereof) are sleek with a very low profile. Although they aren't expensive ($3 U.S.), the lack of padding around the eye pieces makes them less comfortable than those with foam.

The color of goggle lenses varies according to function and fashion. The bright sun reflecting on outdoor pools makes goggles with mirrored or darker lenses a better choice because they block out the harmful UV rays and cut down on glare off the water. However, you'll probably find that when using this same pair of goggles indoors, or for early-morning or late-evening outdoor workouts, when lighting is not as bright, it is difficult to see. Clear or lightly tinted lenses are best in those environments, with a medium tint working well in moderate lighting. Swimmers with less than 20/20 eyesight can order goggles with prescription lenses, but be sure to choose a pair that will fit well to avoid potentially wasting money.

Buying goggles is similar to buying sunglasses. Because shapes of faces and sizes of heads differ from person to person, so will the way goggles fit. Trying them on and playing with the adjustable pieces before purchasing them is a good way to narrow the options, but don't be discouraged or surprised if a return trip or two to the store is necessary before you find the perfect pair. When you do find a pair you're pleased with, buy several in case you can't find them again!

## Swim Cap

Swim caps, though not necessary, are highly recommended in certain cases. Swim caps perform three primary functions that vary in importance depending on the swimmer: protecting hair from chlorine, keeping longer hair out of the face, and reducing drag in the water caused by flowing hair. Swimmers who have little to no hair can focus on their need for speed when deciding whether to wear a cap, as can swimmers whose hair is not adversely affected by chlorine. But most female swimmers, many male swimmers, and nearly all competitive and elite swimmers choose to wear a cap for a combination of its benefits.

Swim caps are constructed primarily of latex or silicone, although Speedo makes a cap with a latex outer surface and Lycra interior. Each type of cap has its advantages and disadvantages. Most competitive swimmers prefer latex caps because they hang onto the head better. The material is stiffer and tighter than silicone, though, so putting them on can be a challenge. Latex caps are also more prone to tears and holes. They can get rubbery over time, especially if left exposed to the sun. Many recreational swimmers wear silicone caps. Silicone is a much more thick and stretchy material than latex, which makes these caps quicker and easier to slide on and off without snagging hair. They last longer than latex caps and offer a more comfortable fit by allowing the head to breathe. However, silicone caps have a tendency

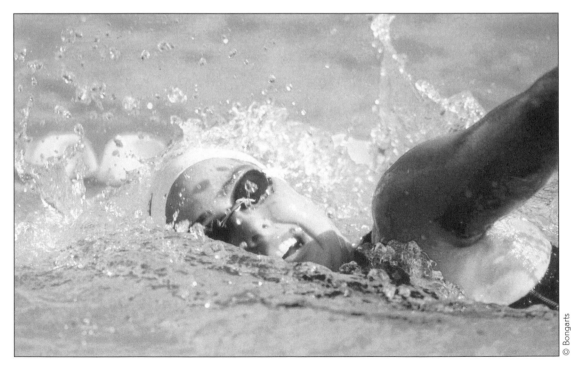

© Bongarts

On my way to gold in the 800-meter freestyle at the 1992 Olympics. Swimming with the proper gear can dramatically improve performance.

to slip off, especially for women. At $7 to $12 U.S. a pair, they can cost up to three or four times the amount of a latex cap, but the longer lifespan probably evens out the expense in the long run.

Chlorine and other pool chemicals tend to make some swimmers' hair develop a faint green tint. A solution to this problem is to put conditioner on the ends of the hair before putting on a cap, which protects hair from the elements of the chlorine. Swimmers who do this tend to prefer latex caps over silicon because the combination of the conditioner and the slippery nature of silicon makes these caps more likely to slide off.

Taking good care of either type of swim cap increases its lifespan. After each workout, dry off the inside and outside of the cap and pat a little talcum powder on the inside to keep it fresh and easier to slip on your head. Depending on how much you swim, a latex cap will last three to four months if you take care of it, and a silicone cap can last up to a year or longer with proper care.

## Towel
I guess a towel falls into the no-brainer category for most swimmers, but so does a swimsuit, so I'll say a few words about towels here, too. Obviously, a towel expedites drying off after swimming—although if you swim outdoors in the summer a towel truly could be considered optional if there's time to dry in the sun. The larger the towel, the more useful it is. A beach towel is easier to wrap around you or sit on if you're lucky enough to have access to a sauna. A beach towel also provides a great surface for preworkout stretching and core-strengthening routines (covered in chapter 4).

## Water Bottle
Submerged in water for most of their training, many swimmers rarely consider dehydration, but they should. In fact, it might be more important to remember to drink fluids during swim workouts for the simple reason that proper hydration is often overlooked. The sensation of sweating is extremely low, if felt at all, when swimming because of the water environment, but swimmers lose fluids through perspiration just as other athletes do.

Have a water bottle near the side of the pool, and sip on it several times during your workout. Drinking up to 16 ounces per hour of swimming should be enough. Unless a workout is extremely challenging or lasts longer than an hour, consuming sport drinks isn't necessary, but go ahead if you think it helps hydration. Generally, though, a workout's duration and energy expenditure doesn't require refueling, so those sports drinks might just be extra calories.

## Log Book
Keeping a log book of your swim workouts, other fitness activities, and, if you compete, races can be extremely beneficial. Regardless of your current fitness level, swimming experience, or length or type of workouts, recording your daily physical activities is motivational and informative because

your progress as a swimmer is laid out in black and white. Although swim-specific log books are available, they are quite small. I've found that a simple notebook works just as well. All but the smallest of notebooks provide more room than most log books, and they cost less. I'll give more details on what to chart in your log book in chapter 3.

## Optional Workout-Enhancing Gear

Once you're clothed and protected for your swim workouts, you might want to consider gear that increases your fitness level by enhancing your workouts. Straight lap swimming is good for your fitness, health, and performance in competition. But a few pieces of additional equipment, focused on specific muscles and technique, might help take you to the next level; their use also goes a long way toward decreasing the potential monotony of a swim workout. Pull buoys, paddles, fins, and kickboards all fall into this category of gear (see figure 1.2). None of them is essential for improved fitness, but all provide substantial gains in performance for the relatively small amount of money they cost. Kickboards are available for use at almost any pool where lap swimming is common. Pull buoys are sometimes available as well, but paddles and fins are more rare, so you'll probably need to buy these yourself. If you choose to use this gear in your workouts regularly, you'll also want to get a bag to tote them in.

The gear discussed in this section will be used in many of the workouts in part II of this book. Some workouts include swimming with pull buoys

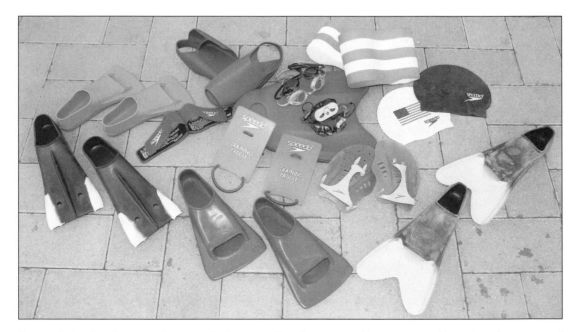

**Figure 1.2** A collection of gear including an MP3 player, an ankle strap, a kickboard, and a variety of fins, paddles, caps, goggles, and pull buoys.

and paddles or kicking with a kickboard or fins. Using proper gear in these workouts helps to develop particular aspects of the stroke or kick, but this doesn't mean the gear is mandatory. In the introduction to part II, I'll explain how to alter your workout if you won't be using one or more pieces of recommended gear.

Using workout-enhancing gear is a good way to make improvements in the pool, but take care not to overdo it. It's easy to get dependent on the aids, especially the fins, because the speed they generate makes swimming more fun. It's necessary to give the body a chance to feel that faster pace in order to get faster, but remember that it's a false speed. Use the gear to build strength, to feel that faster pace, and to spice up a workout, but understand that you won't get the satisfaction of true improvement if you swim with it all the time.

## Pull Buoys and Paddles

Pull buoys provide buoyancy while pulling through the water with the upper body only. Their use improves shoulder strength because the lack of kicking decreases the power of the stroke. A common accoutrement to pull buoys is a pair of paddles, which are worn on the hands to build upper-body strength by increasing the amount of water displaced by the hands during each stroke. Some paddle designs also help retain a feel for the water while working to improve strength. Although pull buoys and paddles can be used separately, it is much more advantageous to use them together.

Pull buoys generally come in one of two shapes. Single-piece buoys are made of a piece of foam somewhat in the shape of an hourglass. Other buoys are made with two identical pieces of cylindrical foam attached by a short piece of nylon rope or strap to form a symmetrical unit in which the round sides of the cylinders are almost touching. Some pull buoys of either shape are made of hollow plastic that can be filled with water; these increase difficulty by decreasing buoyancy and increasing the amount of weight to pull. Using a pull buoy is easy. Simply place the buoy between your thighs and swim with a normal upper-body stroke. Holding the buoy in place prevents almost any kicking while keeping the hips up and the body in a streamline position, which is very important in swimming. Elite swimmers can increase difficulty by putting a stretch band or Velcro strap around their ankles, which prevents even the smallest of kicks from helping propel the body through the water.

Most paddles are made of hard plastic and come in several shapes and sizes. (Some paddles are made of a Lycra-type material and look like gloves with webbed fingers, but I don't recommend these because the cloth-like material gets heavy in the water and can drag the swimmer down.) Most paddles have the shape of a hand, an irregular circle, a square, or a rectangle. Some have holes in them. Each style changes the training focus slightly.

Larger paddles without holes increase strength in the shoulders and arms more dramatically than smaller paddles and paddles with holes do,

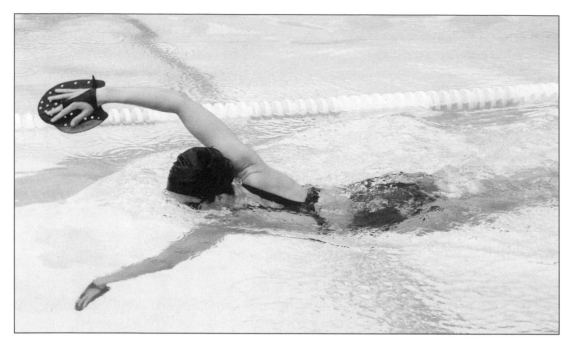

**Figure 1.3**    Training with paddles with holes builds strength and allows a swimmer to retain the feel of the water.

but the primary complaint from elite swimmers about the large, holeless paddles is that they prevent the hands from retaining their feel of the water. Accomplished swimmers know exactly which part of their stroke they're on by the feel of the water on their hands. That awareness is invaluable to performance. When I was competing, I found that if I trained with the large holeless paddles too much, I began to lose my feel for the water and my stroke, and my performance suffered. This is why swim gear manufacturers began to design paddles with holes. The holes reduce the resistance of the paddles but allow swimmers to develop strength while honing and retaining their feel for the water. The benefits are well worth the sacrifice of increased strength, and I recommend choosing paddles with holes in them.

Using paddles too much or too quickly or using paddles that are too large, however, can cause shoulder problems because of the additional strain on the shoulder muscles. The use of any paddle increases speed because of the amount of water moved in each stroke, and because speed is what most swimmers strive to attain, many are tempted to use larger paddles. Smaller swimmers or swimmers just beginning to use paddles should start with a smaller pair to ease the shoulders into the more strenuous workouts. As strength is built, larger paddles can be used safely. Note that regardless of the size of the paddle or the swimmer, distances swum with paddles always should be increased gradually to allow the shoulder muscles to adapt to the effort. The workouts in part II offer guidance on determining safe distances to start with.

# Fins

Fins might be the most enjoyable of all workout equipment because they increase your speed significantly without greatly increasing your workload. Fins can be used alone, in combination with a kickboard, or, if you really want to fly, with paddles. The most common type of fins have rubber blades about 14 to 17 inches (35-43 centimeters) long that are narrow at the foot and build to a width of up to several inches at the tip. Almost every swim gear manufacturer sells these training fins for about $25 U.S. The fins' primary function is to help swimmers move faster through the water. The benefits of doing so are numerous. For one thing, being able to move quickly through the water is motivating. Second, crowded lap swim environments might be easier for slower swimmers with the aid of fins. Third, open-water swimming, especially in an ocean, can be safer with fins because they combat the effects of the waves and currents.

A particular style of fins good for building fitness is called Zoomers, which are shorter but still wide at the toes. Because they don't have the long, flexible rubber helping propel you through the water, Zoomers make the legs work much harder than standard fins do, while still providing an increase in speed. For this reason, Zoomers are a popular training tool to increase leg strength and endurance. When Zoomers are used in combination with paddles, workouts are usually more taxing and burn more calories than normal workouts. Zoomers run about $30 U.S. A recent addition to the swim-fin category is the Z2. Closely related to the Zoomer, the Z2 has a slightly longer blade and increased flexibility, which allows the swimmer to swim at a faster pace but still receive the fitness benefits of the original Zoomer.

Variations of standard fins and Zoomers are also on the market. Some long fins are extra wide at the toe to increase speed, some are notched in the middle to better simulate the flutter kick, and some have varying degrees of flexibility for swimmers with stiff or flexible ankles. The more pliable the fins, the better speed and control they provide. How comfortably the fins fit the heels is important. Fins with heel cups are recommended over fins with heel straps because they offer a better fit. If you plan to use fins extensively, buy a pair one size larger than your shoe size, and wear socks with them to help prevent blisters. You can also purchase "sock shoes" to provide a layer of protection between feet and fins.

In addition to fins meant to be used with the freestyle kick, fins designed to allow simulations of the butterfly and breaststroke kicks are also available. Called a "monofin," this product features a single fin into which both feet are placed. The effect is a dolphin-like kick excellent for practicing the butterfly kick and for strengthening stomach muscles. The high price of monofins (ranging from $50 to $250 U.S.), makes them most attractive to highly competitive swimmers. Fins designed to simulate the breaststroke kick are helpful to swimmers who want to improve that stroke, which is a very technical stroke and difficult to perfect. Again, the price ($40 U.S.) and limited function puts this product in the category of specialty equipment.

## Kickboards

Kickboards help swimmers improve what can be a challenging aspect of swimming. The function of a kickboard is to provide the flotation and support needed to keep the upper body stationary while the lower body propels through the water. Kicking laps is tremendous for building leg strength and endurance and for improving kicking technique.

Swimmers have several options when choosing a kickboard. The most common kickboards are rectangular (about 12 inches [30.5 centimeters] wide and 18 inches [45.7 centimeters] long), have a rounded top, and are made of dense foam. This is the style commonly found at pools. Kickboards of this construction and shape come in different sizes. The smaller the kickboard, the less buoyancy and support it provides, making it more difficult to kick with. Beginning swimmers, those new to kickboards, and those who have great difficulty kicking should start with a large kickboard and progress to smaller sizes as they feel more comfortable kicking. Kickboards also come in a variety of shapes that allow for multiple body and hand positions, but all are very durable. Costs of kickboards range from $7 U.S. for the more basic boards to about $20 U.S. for specialty boards.

## Bags

A bag or two devoted to your life as a swimmer makes things much easier each time you head to the pool, regardless of how much equipment you have. Unless you have a backyard pool, it's almost a given that you'll leave home with a minimum of keys, wallet, cell phone, and towel. Because you will likely also have a change of clothes, goggles, and a swim cap, you'll need a bag unless you want to have several overstuffed pockets.

Manufacturers make swim-specific bags of many shapes and sizes that offer numerous pouches, pockets, and compartments to separate wet gear from dry gear, so there's plenty out there to choose from. Personally, I recommend a mesh bag to carry your pool gear for two reasons. First, your bag containing your valuables should be kept locked in a locker to keep its contents safe and dry, and carting several pieces of gear back and forth from the pool deck to the locker room can be cumbersome. Keeping everything in a mesh bag makes bringing your gear right to the end of your lane convenient. Second, your wet gear will dry much faster in a mesh bag than in a pocket or compartment of a nylon bag.

# Supplemental Gear and Health Aids

These days swim gear can be about as complex as you want to make it. Along with the essentials and a few basic luxuries, there are countless pieces of training gear, health aids, and gadgets that can be used in conjunction with swim workouts. These items vary in importance based on personal preference, but many of them have become quite popular among serious swimmers.

Stretch cords are useful tools in swimming and come in two types. Some are designed to hold the swimmer in one place. The cords are attached at one end to a pole or fence near the edge of the pool, and the other ends are attached to a belt the swimmer wears around the waist. These are useful if there are no lanes dedicated to lap swimming or if the lanes are full but an open swim area is available. Another type of stretch cord can be used for dry-land drills. These cords attach to a pole or solid stationary object; the swimmer holds handles on the other end and performs exercises for stretching, warming up, or strength building. Both types of cords come in different degrees of elasticity, allowing swimmers to alter the difficulty of the workout.

One of the biggest curses of swimming is that it can seem so boring. Runners, walkers, and cyclists are also involved in somewhat monotonous, repetition-filled activities, but their advantage is that their scenery changes. At the pool, you have water and walls. Just as other fitness enthusiasts use music to ward off boredom and take their minds off the task at hand, so can swimmers with underwater MP3 players. These gadgets are not yet perfect in terms of sound quality or function, nor are they appropriate for swimmers who are on a team or who are concentrating on time intervals or sets, but if using an MP3 player will help keep you in the pool, I highly recommend using one.

A nose clip is useful for swimmers who have trouble keeping water out of their noses, but I recommend that only real beginners use a nose clip regularly. The goal should be to get comfortable without one. As I'll explain in the next chapter, one of the secrets of swimming is breathing properly to keep air flowing steadily out of the nose whenever underwater so that no water gets in the passageways. Learning this skill is impossible while wearing a nose clip.

Some swimmers will find certain health aids useful and valuable. Because swimmers are in constant contact with chlorinated water, ocean water, or lake water, products are available to help keep swimmers healthy. Ear plugs enable swimmers to continue swimming while recovering from ear infections. Sunscreen helps prevent skin cancer for outdoor swimmers. Body lotions aid the skin in fighting the drying effects of chlorine. Specialized shampoos and body washes rid the hair of chlorine residue and remove the chlorine smell from the body. Flip-flops help prevent athlete's foot caused by walking on the deck and in the locker room. They also provide easy on-and-off convenience for wet feet after getting out of the pool.

# Swimming Environments

Although swimsuits, goggles, equipment, and health aids are important to swimming, nothing is more necessary than a body of water to swim in. For many swimmers, choices are quite limited. Small towns may have one community pool (and some have none). In colder climates the only pools open year-round are indoors. Swimming in open water is obviously not possible for those living in urban areas with no lakes or oceans nearby.

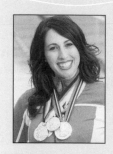

## Circle Patterns Down Under

Although sharing a lane with no more than one other person might be possible for some fitness swimmers, it is not possible for athletes who train with a team or compete in meets where the warm-up pool is crawling with swimmers. Learning to swim circle patterns and become comfortable sharing a lane with several other swimmers is essential. Swimming counterclockwise around a lane became second nature for me, in fact, until I competed in my first international meet in a country in which motorists drive on the left side of the road. A few of my teammates were warming up in the same way that we always did, but suddenly the local swimmers got in and started swimming clockwise. Adjusting was very confusing at first but became a joke among American swimmers who had to watch out for the "crazy drivers" in the pool.

On the other hand, a person living in a large city on the coast in a warm climate might have a plethora of options available, including YMCAs and YWCAs, community centers, aquatic or health clubs, university pools, and lakes or oceans. Regardless of where swimming occurs, certain precautions and points of etiquette should be observed to make swimming safer and more enjoyable for everyone.

## Pools

Swimmers need to be comfortable in the pool they swim in; if they're not, they won't swim as often. Comfort means different things to different people, so look around until you find a pool that makes you want to come back. Shapes and sizes of pools, along with the amenities available in the locker room or fitness center, vary from place to place, but if you're in a medium- to large-sized city, you should be able to find a swimming environment that suits you. If you're in a smaller city, you might need to make the best of what your town offers.

Indoor pools and outdoor pools have the same basic features, but the differing environment they provide each has its pros and cons. An indoor pool is more likely to be open year-round and might be more inviting in the winter in warm climates, when the water in an outdoor pool might be heated but the air temperature is chilly. Chances are, though, an indoor pool will be stuffier, darker, and have a stronger smell of chlorine. An outdoor pool might be more motivating in the summer months, when the weather is sunny and warm, but the weather is not always perfect, and swimmers will have to contend with the elements such as rain and wind. Swimmers who do swim outdoors should always wear sunscreen for protection from skin cancer, even on cloudy or cool days.

The best pools in which to swim for fitness or training are those with lanes or times dedicated to swimming laps. Attempting a serious workout while trying to swim among playing children is difficult, frustrating, and potentially dangerous. Lifeguards on duty should help if children or adults are misusing the lap swim areas when lap swimmers are present. They also might help keep recreational pool users out of a certain area designated for workouts when lap lanes are unavailable.

There are several other optimal characteristics of pools to consider when deciding where to swim. None is vital, but all might enhance your swimming experience and, in some cases, keep you safer. Lane lines—the plastic lane dividers that float on top of the water—and gutters along the edge of the pool keep water turbulence to a minimum and decrease the chance of taking a breath at the same time that a wave arrives at your mouth and nose. Painted or tiled lines at the bottom of the pool in the middle of each lane help swimmers stay on course. The end of those lines, sometimes marked with a perpendicular line to form the shape of a T, are useful in helping swimmers know when to begin executing a flip turn. A row of small triangular flags hanging above the pool indicate to backstrokers how far they are from the end of the lane.

Many, if not most, pools have at least one clock on the pool deck or wall called a pace clock. (For instruction on how to read and use a pace clock, see chapter 3.) If the pool you choose does not have a pace clock, purchase a waterproof digital watch to wear during your workouts. A pace clock is preferable, but a watch will allow you to time your workouts, which typically brings greater improvement, as explained in chapter 3.

Among pools with lap lanes and dedicated lap swim times, the distances of those lanes can vary significantly. However, there are two common lengths of pools that mirror those used in competition. The more common length in the United States, referred to in competition as "short course," is 25 yards (22.8 meters) long. A "long-course" pool is 50 meters (54.6 yards) long. Swimming in a long-course pool will increase fitness levels more quickly and significantly because swimmers don't get that extra break or boost off the wall at 25 yards that shorter pools afford. As you might expect, swimming in 50-meter pools is much more challenging, especially for newer swimmers. Long-course pools are also more difficult to find, however, so the workouts in this book are based on the short-course length. (Adjusting times or distances will be necessary if your regular pool is of a longer or shorter length; how to make such adjustments is discussed in the introduction to part II.)

A particular etiquette is expected in lap swimming. Some pools have posted rules to follow that keep lap swim sessions more organized and allow for a greater number of swimmers to safely and comfortably participate.

Even if your pool doesn't have posted rules, the following points of etiquette should be followed in any lap swim situation.

- **Choose the right lane speed.** During lap swim times, many pools have lanes designated for slower, medium, and faster swimmers, but not all pools do. Choose the lane in which swimmers are closest in speed to yours. Don't overestimate your speed. If necessary, time the swimmers in each lap to assess where you fit in.

- **Be considerate when joining someone in a lane.** Don't stop a swimmer in the middle of a swim set or interval. Wait until he or she has stopped to ask if you may split the lane.

- **When only two people are sharing a lane, swimmers should stay on their own sides.** Sharing a lane is sometimes stressful for newer swimmers and for those who have difficulty swimming in a straight line. By being aware of any straying tendencies and the location of your lane mate, as well as focusing on your distance from the lane line at all times, any anxiety of sharing a lane will be minimized and decrease with practice.

- **When two or more people are sharing a lane, swimmers should swim in a circle pattern.** In countries in which cars travel in the right lane, such as the United States, the circle pattern is counterclockwise, so the swimmer always stays on the right-hand side of the pool. In countries in which cars travel in the left lane, such as Great Britain, Australia, and Japan, the circle pattern is clockwise, so the swimmer always stays on the left-hand side of the pool. Swimmers must be very conscious of other swimmers in their lane. Adjustments will likely need to be made in speed and swimming sets, and care should be taken when passing swimmers to prevent collisions or the disrupting of another swimmer's rhythm. Swimming circle patterns is difficult, and it takes time to become comfortable doing so. Circle patterns are not ideal, especially for interval workouts, but sometimes they are unavoidable. The skill of swimming circle patterns is also developed with experience.

- **Be considerate of other people's workout routines.** If someone is in the middle of an interval set, don't strike up a conversation with him or her. Interrupting an athlete in the middle of a bench press is unheard of, and so should be interrupting someone in the middle of a swim set.

- **Return any borrowed equipment to its holding place.** Do not leave community gear lying at the end of your lane after a workout thinking someone else might want to use it later. Keep the swim deck uncluttered.

When all's said and done, the best pool for you is the one you enjoy going to and to which you want to return. Swimmers with limited choices are wise to make the best of their situation or join a committee to work on improving their facility choices. Because swimming in a community pool will almost always cost money, swimmers with options are advised to shop around

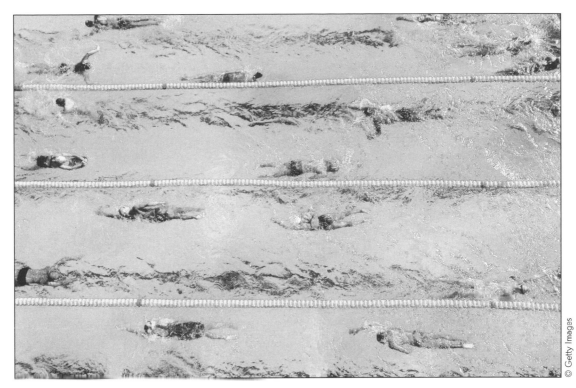

© Getty Images

The counterclockwise circle pattern is used when many swimmers must share a lane, such as during a precompetition warm-up session.

until they find the environment that best suits their needs and preferences before joining a particular gym or center.

## Open-Water Swimming

Swimming in a lake or ocean can be exciting and adventurous and can add some spice to your workouts. But open-water swimming is very different from swimming in a pool, and being aware of certain dangers and tendencies of open-water swimming will help keep you and others safe. The safest way to swim in open water is to swim with someone. Informing others of your plan (particularly those closest in relationship and proximity to you) is also smart, as is letting any lifeguard on duty know what you are doing.

Two aspects of swimming in open water make it especially difficult to keep a straight course: the lack of lane lines and the currents (especially in an ocean). Stop swimming periodically and alter your direction accordingly. Even if your form keeps you swimming in a straight line, subtly strong currents and waves might throw you off course. Also, weather can change very quickly, especially on a large body of water. Swimming laps near your base is wise in case conditions grow unfavorable or you begin to feel unexpectedly tired or sick.

Proper equipment is important when swimming in open water. I strongly recommend that beginning open-water swimmers wear large fins to help them deal with currents and waves. All open-water swimmers should make sure their gear works before getting too far from base. Swimming a few times in a pool before heading to open water will help get you used to the gear and ensure that it fits and works properly. In a pool you're never more than 50 meters or yards away from your base or a short distance away from the edge, but in an ocean, making adjustments is much more difficult. Common sense and some planning are crucial to your safety when swimming in open water.

# chapter 2

# Stroke and Turn Technique

Stroke technique is the cornerstone of fast, efficient swimming. Beginning fitness swimmers, accomplished masters swimmers, and elite competitors alike should focus each workout on refining their technique. Even the best swimmers in the world constantly work on their strokes. Without good technique, the chances of improvement in swimming diminish significantly. The instruction in this chapter is thorough yet concise and will be helpful to those fairly new to swimming, swimmers proficient at one or two strokes but not all four, and experienced swimmers, who can always use a review of the key elements of stroke execution that will help them improve. In this chapter I'll first discuss the general techniques that pertain to any stroke and then cover the techniques of the freestyle, backstroke, breaststroke, and butterfly. The chapter concludes with a discussion of turns—the flip turn used in freestyle and the backstroke as well as the turn employed in the breaststroke and butterfly.

## General Swimming Techniques

A few concepts in swimming hold true regardless of the stroke being used. The first, and perhaps most obvious of these is that swimmers should breathe out only while underwater and breathe in only while above the surface. Second, the core muscles of the body should be flexed throughout every stroke or position while swimming. Third, the streamline position puts the body in the most efficient position to move through the water and should be employed to some degree on virtually every lap. Finally, stroke efficiency is a delicate, individualized balance of stroke count, stroke length, and stroke rate.

# Breathing

The most important aspect of swimming is breathing. Swimmers who can't breathe properly in the water can't work effectively on anything else. Swimming is like yoga, Pilates, or scuba diving in that breathing plays a key role. Proper breathing eventually becomes second nature, but until it does it must be emphasized and practiced continually.

The beauty of breathing in the water is its simplicity. Whenever the face is underwater, breaths should be exhaled steadily through the nose. The mouth should be closed but relaxed. Whenever the face is above water, breaths should be inhaled through the mouth. That's really all there is to breathing while swimming and feeling comfortable in the water, but of course in the beginning it's not as easy as it sounds. Some beginning swimmers panic when they get underwater and wind up doing one of two things. A beginner might hold her breath underwater, which tightens up the body and causes it to sink. This mistake also makes for a very busy second or two when she comes up for air because she will try to get all of the breathing done at once—in and out and in and out—before putting her head back in the water. The other tendency is to exhale through the mouth but then breathe in through the nose, which, of course, gets water in the nose. Neither result is conducive to becoming more comfortable in the water.

Blowing out through the nose also applies when diving into the water or doing flip turns. For some reason, many young swimmers forget to breathe out when doing flip turns and wind up with water up their noses. Essentially, if you're not blowing out, you're either holding your breath, which isn't good, or you're breathing in, which is worse.

To get comfortable underwater and to develop the habit of breathing out underwater and breathing in above water, try pretending you're a child blowing bubbles underwater. Hang on to the edge of the pool or stand in water no higher than the chest. Take a deep breath, put your whole body underwater, and blow as much of the air out as possible through your nose. Come back up, take another deep breath, and then go down and do it again. This little exercise might feel juvenile, but it remains the best way to get comfortable with breathing.

# Core Stability

Have you every wondered why elite swimmers have such great stomach muscles? It is because no matter what their stroke or distance specialty, their core muscles—those in the abdomen, back, and hips—are doing a huge amount of work in the water. Everything in swimming starts with the core. Balance comes from the abdomen, which is the center of a swimmer's world in the pool. Abdominal and back muscles are constantly working to keep the limbs stretched out, and all 29 of the core muscles work in cooperation to keep the body in the streamline position. Because the core is so important to swimming, and because everyone can benefit from toning and strengthening their core muscles, chapter 4 includes seven exercises for the core that aid not only swimming but also posture, balance, and control on dry land.

# Streamline Position

Cruise liners, kayaks, and fish have at least one thing in common. Their design puts them in position to travel most efficiently through water. The design of airplanes and birds provides the same effect for their journeys through air. Moving through water is more difficult than moving through air or on land, so the need to be energy efficient is heightened in an aquatic environment. Although extraneous movement should be avoided in any sport or activity in which conserving energy is beneficial, even more care should be given to remaining in as hydrodynamic a position as possible in water because water presents so much more resistance. The position that allows swimmers to move through the water most quickly and efficiently is called the *streamline position*.

In the streamline position, the body is horizontal to the bottom of the pool, belly down, and stretched out as long as possible. Both arms are straight and extended in front of the head, with shoulders pressed against the ears and one hand on top of the other. Legs are straight and extended behind the body, and ankles and toes point away from the body (figure 2.1).

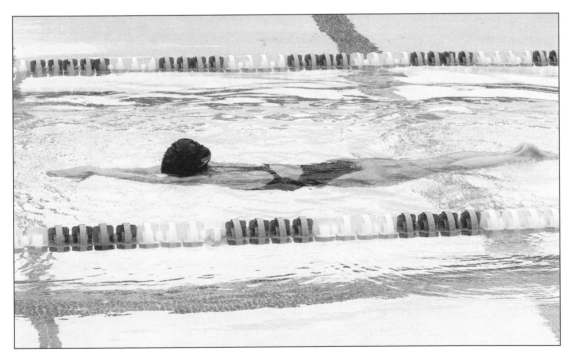

**Figure 2.1** Proper technique in the streamline position reduces drag, allowing the swimmer to move through the water quickly and efficiently.

Swimmers assume a streamline position to make the smallest possible profile in the water, which keeps the drag created by the body at a minimum. Moving a flat hand through the water when the palm is perpendicular to the bottom of the pool is more difficult than moving a flat hand through the water when the palm is parallel to the bottom of the pool because the profile of the hand is smaller. If the trunk of the body remains aligned behind the arms and if the hips and legs remain aligned behind the trunk, the profile of the body moving through the water is only as wide as the widest point of the body and as deep as the depth of the trunk.

The most common mistake is allowing the hips and legs to drop out of alignment and sink below the trunk. When this happens, the body's profile increases dramatically. Instead of a torpedo-shaped body cutting through the water, a V-shaped body is being dragged through the water. Keeping the stomach muscles flexed and adding a slight kick helps keep the body in proper alignment.

Each of the four strokes in swimming uses the streamline position to varying degrees. The body is most often in the streamline position or a variation thereof in the freestyle and backstroke. But with every push off the wall, regardless of the upcoming stroke, the body should be streamlined to achieve maximum distance through minimum effort. The thrust off the wall provides momentum; the streamline position provides efficiency. After a swimmer pushes off the wall and assumes a streamline position, a small flutter or butterfly kick helps the body stay balanced and prolongs the optimal use of the streamline before the stroke is commenced. The benefit of moving streamlined through the water after pushing off from the wall is the brief rest the body receives while still moving forward at a decent speed. Speed soon decreases to a point at which it no longer makes sense to glide through the water. How long the streamline position should be retained after the push off the wall varies for each swimmer and is based on the answers to several questions. How strong is the swimmer's push? How efficiently does the swimmer glide through the water? What is the swimmer's goal for the particular lap, set, race, or workout being swum?

## Stroke Efficiency

The number of strokes it takes to swim from one end of the pool to the other (stroke count) depends on how far each stroke moves the body forward in the water (stroke length) and how quickly the strokes come (stroke frequency, stroke rate, tempo, or turnover). More important, though, than the individual factors in determining the speed at which a swimmer crosses a pool is stroke efficiency. For instance, if a swimmer with long but slow strokes raced against a swimmer with quick but short strokes, it would be impossible to determine based on that information alone who would win the race. The efficiency of each swimmer's stroke must also be known.

The key to swimming faster is to pull as much water as possible with each stroke. The amount of water that can possibly be pulled depends on a swimmer's size and muscle mass. Quick strokes that don't move the body very far aren't effective in producing speed. The swimmer is basically spinning his or her wheels, like the cartoon character who starts to run but doesn't go anywhere. The arms are rotating quickly, but there's no clean catch of the water at the top of the underwater stroke and no strong push at the hips to end the stroke. Conversely, speed will suffer if you take long, stretched-out strokes with slow turnover.

There is no one best stroke count, stroke length, or stroke frequency. If all stroke efficiency were equal, a shorter swimmer would always require a higher turnover rate to maintain the pace of a taller swimmer. That is not the case. A swimmer with a strong pull won't need as high a stroke count as a swimmer who moves less water with each stroke. The key is to develop the most efficient combination of stretch, frequency, and count for your body and strengths and then to focus on mastering that stroke in training. Some swimmers get in a comfortable groove and stretch out very well on each stroke but develop a slow tempo in the process; others try to match someone

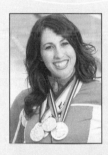

## Stroke Count

Conventional wisdom, common sense, and historical fact all point to the high probability that a swimmer with greater height and longer arms will outswim a shorter swimmer with shorter arms. But the women's 400-meter freestyle competition at the 1988 Olympic Games in Seoul, South Korea, provided an excellent illustration of the importance of stroke efficiency and the relative lack of importance of a lower stroke count.

At 5 feet 3 inches, I was short by swimmer standards and quite short compared to the East Germans lined up next to me for the 400-meter freestyle. Because I had always been smaller than my competitors, I had learned early on that the fastest way for me to get to the other end of the pool was to move my arms as quickly as possible. That produced a very high stroke count, which is generally considered a bad idea. But through continual work on my technique I was able to maximize my stroke efficiency by achieving excellent rotation in my hips and shoulders, a clean catch, and a strong push from my hips to the end of my stroke.

The focus in swim training often is on lowering stroke count to increase speed, and that tactic is solid as long as efficiency is not lost. My stroke count was quite high—about 40 strokes per 50 meters compared to 25 for the larger swimmers—but my strong pull and push underwater and rapid tempo combined to create an efficient stroke that earned me a gold medal against the larger swimmers in that 400-meter freestyle race.

else's frequency and start spinning out a bit. There's a fine line to finding a natural balance, but once found it makes a world of difference. The distance to be swum also plays a role in determining the most efficient stroke. Stroke technique doesn't change, but tempo does. A really fast tempo with good underwater technique can wear a swimmer out quickly. The goal is to find a comfortable stroke rate that coincides with the distance to be swum.

# Stroke-Specific Techniques

Most fitness swimmers and triathletes swim freestyle almost exclusively, and the number of freestyle events at most meets is about double that for other strokes. Freestyle is usually the stroke that's learned first and thus the most comfortable and natural for most swimmers. That said, in this section we'll cover all four strokes, not just the freestyle, for two reasons. First, the fitness benefits of each stroke are a little different. Second, some of the workouts in chapters 5 through 9 incorporate all four strokes to add interest and variety into your swimming regimen.

## Freestyle

When someone mentions swimming, the image that usually comes to mind is the freestyle stroke. The freestyle is the fastest stroke, it is used in more events than any other at swim meets, it is the easiest of the strokes to learn, and it is generally the first stroke a swimmer learns. In this section we'll look at the four primary features of the freestyle stroke: body and head position, upper-body movement, kicking, and breathing.

### Body and Head Position

As is true for all strokes, the freestyle stroke starts with the core muscles. The lower abdominal muscles are flexed to keep the hips high in the water. The upper and side abdominal muscles are working to constantly rotate the body. The back muscles are lending support to the arms.

The freestyle stroke begins in the streamline position after the push off the wall, with the body stretched out as long as it can be, one hand on top of the other, belly parallel to the bottom of the pool, and hips aligned with the trunk. As the swimmer moves through the water, the body should rotate on an axis, which shifts the position of the swimmer's belly in relation to the bottom of the pool—it doesn't remain parallel. Imagine a swimmer standing on a pool deck with a pole running straight through her body. The pole enters the body in the middle of the top of the head and runs through the neck and the middle of the trunk (figure 2.2). Now imagine that swimmer in the water in streamline position. The imaginary pole acts as an axis on which a swimmer's shoulders, torso, hips, and legs rotate.

The body turns 180 degrees for each stroke, or 90 degrees to each side from center. As the left hand enters the water, the shoulders, body, and hips should begin turning clockwise. By the time the arm is fully extended and just before it begins pulling, the body should be at a 90-degree angle facing the right side of the pool. Then, as the left arm is pulling and the right arm is moving overhead (figure 2.3), the body begins to rotate counterclockwise so that, by the time the right arm is fully extended and just before it begins pulling, the body will be at a 90-degree angle facing the left side of the pool. We call this position—in which one arm is fully stretched in front of the body, the other arm is fully stretched behind the body, and the body is facing either the left or the right side of the pool—the extended position (figure 2.4). As you can see, the angle of the body in relation to the bottom of the pool is never static but instead is constantly turned either 90 degrees to the right or left. After the pushoff, the only time a swimmer's belly is exactly parallel to the bottom of the pool is that precise moment between rotating from one side to the other.

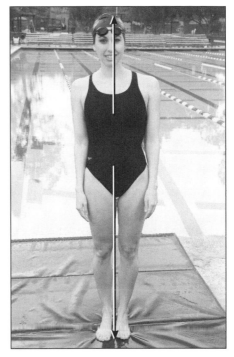

**Figure 2.2** In the freestyle stroke, a swimmer's body rotates on an imaginary axis.

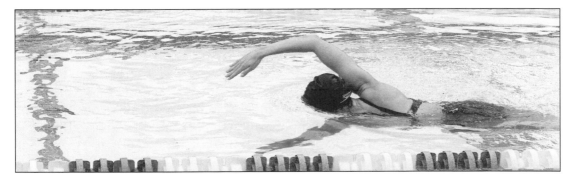

**Figure 2.3** As the left arm begins pulling, the body begins to rotate counterclockwise.

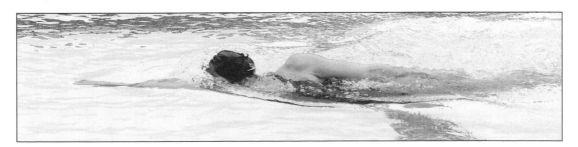

**Figure 2.4** The extended freestyle position, with both arms fully stretched and the body at a 90-degree angle.

The head position should be relaxed, with the water striking the forehead somewhere between the hairline (depending on where your hairline is) and the top of the eyebrows. The head shouldn't be so far under that the eyes must stare at the bottom of the pool. Nor should the neck be so flexed that it lifts the eyes or face out of the water. A natural, neutral posture leads the rest of the body into the streamline position.

## Upper-Body Movement

The fingertips should enter the water at about a 45-degree angle. Hands are relaxed, a tiny space separates the fingers, and the thumb is at ease and pointing in the same direction as the fingers. The finger and thumb positions are similar to that of a friendly wave. This position is called the catch. Some swimmers' fingers and thumb are in a high-five position; they slap the water forcefully, as if they're trying to hit the bottom of the pool. Other swimmers cup their hands and enter the water timidly, as if to avoid making a splash. Neither method allows swimmers to get any pull in the water as they begin their stroke. The goal is a clean catch; the movement of the hand toward the body should create no bubbles. Bubbles indicate that air is present in front of the palm. Any air in front of the palm displaces what could be more water that the hand is moving. Thus, bubbles signify lack of efficiency in the stroke.

Each stroke should begin with arms fully extended, but that doesn't mean the hand enters the water in that position. The arms should not be thrown into the water as far away from the head as possible. The hand should slice the water at a natural, comfortable distance in front of the head. As the arm stretches forward, use the body's flexibility and rotation on the axis to achieve maximum reach.

After the forward arm enters the water and the body is stretched into the extended position, apply pressure to the water with the fingertips and palm. That motion automatically causes the hand to begin moving into a position perpendicular to the bottom of the pool, which forces the elbow to rise. This marks the beginning of the pull phase of the stroke. The power of the stroke comes from the forearm, hand, and biceps leveraging against the elbow to pull water toward the body. Some swimmers begin the pull phase as if they were holding a doorknob and pulling a door toward them. This causes the elbow to lead the stroke and negates the power of the elbow when it acts as a fulcrum. As the pull begins, with the elbow still underwater, the hand begins to move in the shape of a backward S—away from the body and toward the wall of the pool about 12 to 15 inches (30-38 centimeters) before turning in and heading toward the hip. Once the hand nearly reaches the hip bone, it turns back away from the body to finish the backward S and the stroke. Remember to lead with the fingertips, palm, and forearm; let the elbow simply follow (figure 2.5).

The consistent rotation of the shoulders while swimming freestyle creates mirrored arm actions similar to a seesaw. The arms are always opposite of

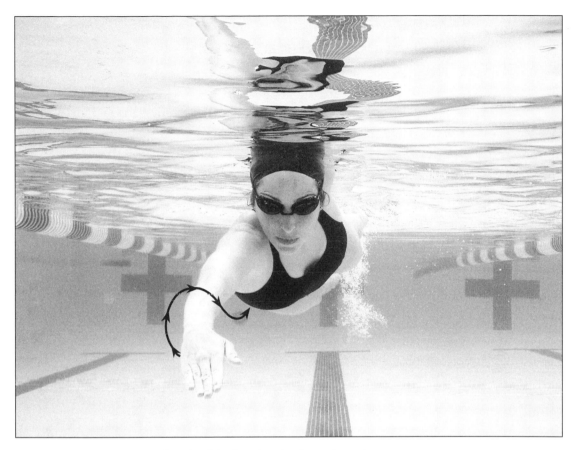

**Figure 2.5**   The backward-S path of the hand in the freestyle stroke.

each other, with the head acting as the fulcrum. When one arm moves in front of the head above the water, the other arm begins to push past the hips below the water. When the right arm is stretching, the left arm is pushing, and both arms finish at the same time. When the arms are in the extended position, the forward arm is ready to begin the pull, and the back arm is exiting the water. In addition to the imaginary pole serving as an axis on which the body rotates, there is also an imaginary line that bisects the body, splitting the forehead, nose, and bellybutton and extending above the head an arm's length. The hands and arms should never cross that line. The left hand should enter and exit the water on the left side of the body, and the right hand should enter and exit the pool on the right side of the body.

The freestyle recovery is what the arm does above the water. While one arm is underwater, the other arm is in recovery as it moves above the water from the end of its previous stroke to the beginning of its next stroke. The recovery should be a natural motion for the swimmer. The most common arm position during recovery is a bent elbow. Bending the elbow keeps the shoulder from having to make a complete revolution in its socket.

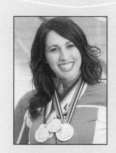

# Freestyle Recovery

Old-school swimming philosophies and most technique books maintain the importance of bending the elbow when the arm is in recovery. That technique is probably the prettiest to watch, and it saves the shoulders from making a complete rotation every stroke. However, my recovery was different. I didn't bend my elbows. People used to make fun of my straight-arm recovery, and maybe they still do despite my long career as a distance freestyler.

What my success taught me was that it really doesn't matter what your arm does above the water. You can bend your elbow. You can keep your arm straight. You can wave to your mom in the stands if you want. The important thing is to get your hand back in the water in perfect position to start your pull.

I don't necessarily recommend that beginning swimmers learn the straight-arm recovery, but I do suggest a relaxed version of the bent-elbow recovery rule. I think that each swimmer should choose the degree to which the elbow bends and the shoulder revolves. At the end of the day, if your arm is more straight than bent, it makes little difference. What matters in swimming fast is what's happening underneath the water.

## Kicking

The kick might be the second-most difficult aspect of swimming. For all strokes, the kick helps keep the body in optimal position and provides both power and balance. The kicking action in the freestyle comes mostly from the hips and ankles. Many swimmers feel they must bend their knees to 90-degree angles to swim freestyle. But, really, the feet and knees should stay quite relaxed, not locked tight and stiff but loose and at ease. The bulk of the power should come from the hip muscles, quadriceps, and hamstrings.

Initiate the kick with the hips, alternately moving the legs up and down about six inches (15 centimeters) and allowing the relaxed ankles to flop in the water, which makes for a full transfer of the energy in the legs into the water. This action keeps the hips up and the body moving forward. The feet should stay underwater for the most part, with the heels occasionally breaking the surface (figure 2.6). The greater the flexibility in the ankles, the more force exerted against the water. The result of a proper kick is to keep the hips in streamline position and provide propulsion through the water. If the kick isn't executed correctly, the hips and legs will sink even if the abdominal muscles are flexed and doing their job.

Most problems with the kick begin with three common mistakes. One, swimmers bend their knees too much, which uses up energy before it's released into the water through the ankle. Overbent knees also create more surface of the body that must cut through the water. Two, swimmers either

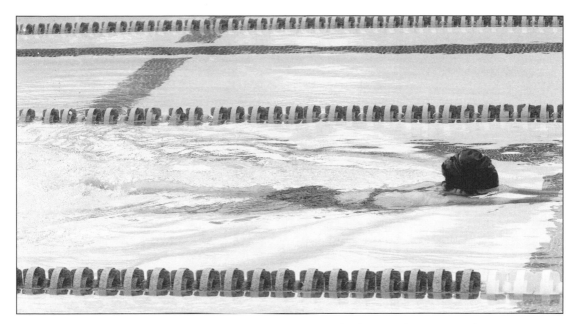

**Figure 2.6** In the freestyle kick, the knees are relaxed and the feet mostly remain underwater.

drop their hips or, in an effort to keep from doing so, overcorrect by raising their hips. Either way takes the body out of streamline position and creates extra work. Three, the swimmer overkicks. This deprives the body of much-needed oxygen, causing the hips and legs to fatigue too quickly and to sink in the water. Fitness swimmers who find themselves kicking all the time are probably doing so because their legs are sinking and they're trying to keep them up.

Kicking should be relaxed and rhythmic. The rhythm is generally determined by the distance the swimmer normally swims. There are three common rhythms to the freestyle kick.

- **Six-beat kick.** In a six-beat kick, the legs are kicking throughout the entire stroke cycle, which consists of one full stroke of both arms. At no point do the legs stop kicking, which averages out to about six kicks per stroke cycle. Most sprinters use a six-beat kick because their goal is to generate as much speed as possible for a short duration.

- **Four-beat kick.** In a four-beat kick, the legs are kicking during each stroke cycle but take a very brief break during each breath, which averages out to about four kicks per cycle. Middle-distance swimmers use this rhythm to give their legs a break.

- **Two-beat kick.** In a two-beat kick, a leg kicks once for every arm stroke. This rhythm is the least tiring and is a natural preference for many fitness swimmers. I recommend this rhythm for fitness swimmers for the same reason that it's the choice of most elite distance swimmers: It allows you to swim for longer distances because less oxygen is diverted to the legs.

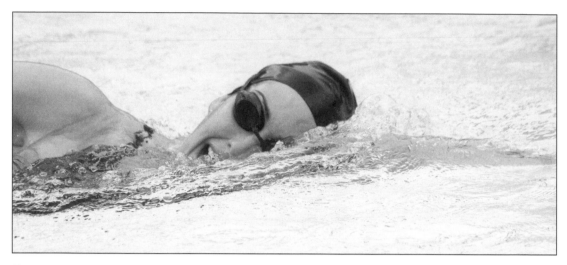

**Figure 2.7**  To take a freestyle breath, turn the face to the side as the body moves through the extended position.

## Breathing

The two methods of breathing for the freestyle stroke are single-sided breathing and alternate breathing. Single-sided breathing is when every breath is taken on the same side of the body, either the left or the right. Alternate breathing is when breaths are taken on alternating sides of the body. Single-sided breathing is much easier than alternate breathing but tends to create a dominant side of the swimmer. Single-sided breathers generally take a breath every second or fourth stroke. Alternate breathers tend to breathe every third or fifth stroke. The benefit of alternate breathing is that it keeps the swimmer's body more balanced in strength and stability.

To breathe on the right side, turn the face to the right, placing the left ear against the left shoulder as the right arm leaves the water (figure 2.7). Inhale quickly, and as the right arm makes its way over the head and the left arm moves behind the body, turn the head back into the proper head position. The eyes should be looking at the side of the pool when it's time to take a breath.

It's not necessary to open the mouth wide to get a breath. Open the side of the mouth that is away from the water to draw in air, leaving the side of the mouth closest to the water closed to keep water out. Some swimmers open their mouths really wide, as if they're visiting a dentist, but that isn't necessary. A half-open mouth can take in enough air to last until the next breath.

## Backstroke

The concepts of the backstroke are similar to those of the freestyle. The fundamental difference is obviously that the freestyle is swum on the belly and the backstroke is swum on the back. The two major similarities are the importance of staying in streamline position and the rotation of the body on an axis. Because of the similarities of the two strokes, swimmers often pick up the techniques of the backstroke best when it's introduced immediately after the freestyle.

The backstroke employs the lower-abdominal muscles that hold up the hips and legs as well as the upper and side muscles used to create the rotation on the axis. The bonus benefit, for some swimmers, is that the face is generally out of the water, making breathing much easier.

## Body and Head Position

Other than being flip-flopped, the positions of the body and head in the backstroke are exactly like those in freestyle, using the streamline position. The head is neutral and relaxed, yet it should stay perfectly straight throughout the stroke. The chin should not be tucked to the collarbone; the neck should not be flexed so that the chin rises and points upward. The body follows in alignment behind the head, with the trunk, hips, and legs all staying on the same plane. This keeps the body profile small and drag low. One problem some swimmers have with the backstroke is they tend to relax their abdominal muscles, which allows the hips and bottom to sink. This puts the swimmer's body in almost a V shape, increasing the surface area of the body that must move through water.

Backstrokers swim with the same imaginary pole serving as the axis on which their bodies rotate. The 180-degree rotation with each stroke allows for the longest reach and most powerful stroke possible. The extended position of the freestyle also applies to the backstroke. When watching world-class backstrokers swim away from the cameras during a televised competition, that position of stretching and rotation is easy to see. Watch for the way these swimmers get their shoulders up to their chins with each stroke.

A fun yet effective way to feel the similarities of the body position and rotation in the backstroke and the freestyle is the Corkscrew Drill. Take one freestyle stroke with the right arm, rotating from streamline position 90 degrees clockwise. Then, instead of rotating 180 degrees counterclockwise for the next freestyle stroke, rotate another 180 degrees clockwise. This puts you on your back and in position for your next stroke to be a backstroke stroke with the left arm. Continue swimming in this corkscrew manner to the end of the lane. On the return lap, corkscrew the opposite direction, with a left-arm freestyle stroke leading into a right-arm backstroke stroke.

## Upper-Body Movement

The hand is in that same relaxed, friendly wave position when it enters the water, but the pinkie side of the hand enters the water first in a choplike motion. The arm is stretched straight out from the body in line with the shoulder (figure 2.8). When the pinkie leads the hand into the water (instead of the back of the hand hitting the water first), the hand is in perfect position to begin the stroke. There's no need to adjust hand position underwater, which wastes time and energy.

The 180-degree rotation isn't complete when the pinkie hits the water. Because the arms stay exactly opposite each other as they do in freestyle, the hand finishing the stroke should be leaving the water when the pinkie of the hand beginning the stroke enters the water. The body isn't able to finish that 180-degree rotation, opening up to its fullest length, until the hand finishing a stroke leaves the water.

The pinkie, hand, and arm should enter the water with enough force to provide the initial momentum for moving down and into the fully stretched position. The extension of the forward arm is happening as it lowers into the water, whereas in freestyle the extension continues in that streamline position. Once the arm in the water is fully extended, bend the elbow in about a 20-degree angle to initiate the catch, or the pull phase of the stroke. Pull the hand toward the rib cage, leading with the elbow (figure 2.9). By the time the elbow touches the bottom part of the back side of the rib cage, the elbow should be at a 90-degree angle to provide maximum strength in the push phase of the stroke. Bringing the hand closer to the hips and rib cage, push the water past the hips (figure 2.10). This is the real power position of the stroke, created by that elbow bend just as it is in the freestyle.

Because the seesaw action of the arms holds true in backstroke, the arm beginning its stroke should enter the water and move toward and past the hips below water as the other arm leaves the water, palm down, and moves

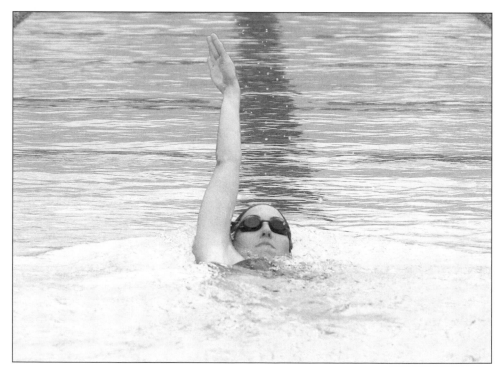

**Figure 2.8** Approaching the backstroke entry, with the pinkie leading the hand into the water.

toward and past the hips above water. As the arm above water makes its way up the body in preparation to begin a new stroke, the arm and hand slowly and naturally rotate so that the pinkie side is ready to lead the hand into the water. Like freestylers, backstrokers have an imaginary line running up the spine and extending an arm's length above the head. The hands should never cross that line at any point during the stroke, especially as they enter the water.

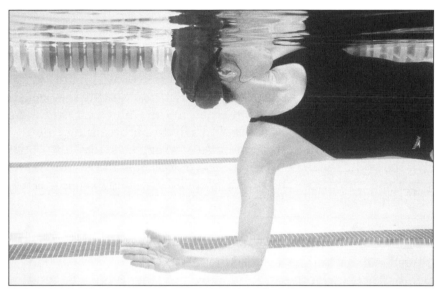

**Figure 2.9** The pull phase of the backstroke.

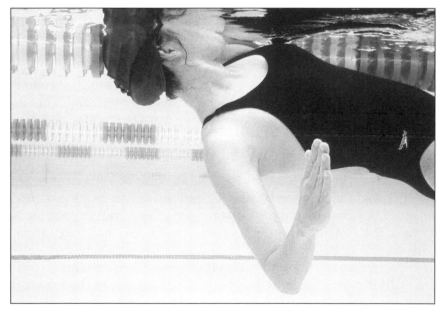

**Figure 2.10** The push phase of the backstroke.

## Kicking

The backstroke kick is the same as the freestyle kick. The kick originates in the hips, and power is transferred down through relaxed legs and ankles and to the water through the feet. The common problem in the kick when swimming either freestyle or backstroke is the knee bend. Seeing and correcting that flaw is much easier when swimming backstroke because the knees come directly out of the water. You never want to look down during the backstroke and see the knees bending at 90-degree angles as if you're riding a bicycle on your back.

## Breathing

Breathing is easier in the backstroke than in any other stroke. Because the face is virtually always out of the water, backstrokers can breathe whenever they want. That's not to say the face doesn't get wet during the backstroke, because it does, but it's never submerged in the water as it is in the other three strokes. Even so, it's best to develop a rhythmic breathing pattern—out through the nose and in with the mouth—to keep a steady flow of oxygen entering the body. The benefit of the backstroke is that the rhythm is entirely the swimmer's preference and doesn't depend on when the mouth and nose are out of the water.

# Breaststroke

The breaststroke is unique because the upper body and lower body work independently of each other, although the movements must be coordinated to begin and end at the same time. In the freestyle and backstroke, the timing is keyed off of where the hands are in relation to the rest of the body, and the rotation of the shoulders, torso, and hips are interrelated. In the breaststroke, the arms are doing one thing and the legs are doing another, but the two separate actions are executed in unison.

The movements of the breaststroke develop excellent core muscles along the entire back and abdominal area, increase flexibility of the back and quadriceps, and strengthen the leg muscles. Because of the leg actions during the kicking phase, the efficiency of the breaststroke is enhanced by good flexibility of the quadriceps, knees, and ankles.

## Body and Head Position

The core muscles in both the back and the abdominals are worked significantly when swimming breaststroke. The lower and midback muscles keep the hips and bottom up, and the upper and midback muscles lift the upper body out of the water during each stroke. The abdominals flex to keep the body in streamline position.

The breaststroke begins with the body in a modified streamline position, the only difference being the placement of the hands. In the breaststroke, the arms are rotated inward so that the backs of the hands are facing each other and the palms face the sides of the pool (figure 2.11).

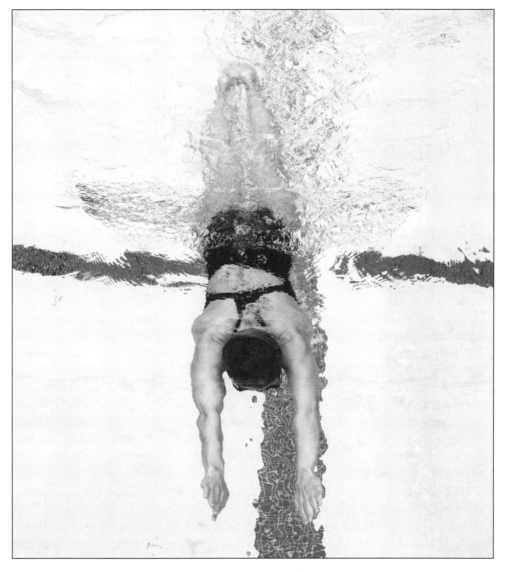

**Figure 2.11**  The modified streamline position in the breaststroke.

The head position in relation to the shoulders should remain constant throughout the breaststroke, although its position in relation to the water will change during the stroke's various phases. During the first half of the stroke cycle, the head is in streamline position. During the last half of the stroke cycle, the head, shoulders, and upper body rise out of the water at about a 45-degree angle, with the head in that natural streamline position in relation to the upper body. When the head returns to the water, the eyes should be staring at the bottom of the pool before the head gradually returns to the streamline position and the swimmer begins the pull and prepares to bring the face out of the water for a breath.

## Upper-Body Movement

The movement of the arms during the breaststroke is best learned through imagery. Picture a large bowl sitting just underneath the water's surface. When in the modified streamline position, the near edge of the bowl sits just in front of the chin, and the far edge is at the fingertips. The diameter of the bowl is about twice the swimmer's shoulder width, extending about half the width of the shoulders on each side of the body. Along the edge of the bowl is your favorite cake batter. The motion of the arms and hands during the breaststroke is as if you were gathering as much batter as you can in your fingertips and palms from the edge of the bowl.

From the modified streamline position, the arms begin to separate as the fingertips and palms move along the lip inside of the imaginary bowl. For the first few inches (or the first dozen centimeters), the arms remain straight, but for the fingertips to continue following the circle shape of the bowl, the elbows must bend. Take care not to form a V above the bowl by continuing to keep the arms straight as you begin to pull the water. Bending those elbows helps the hands follow along the edge of the circumference of the bowl (figure 2.12a).

When hands and forearms are near the bottom of the bowl and are about shoulder-width apart, the elbows should be bent tightly in about 90-degree angles and squeezed into the body. The forearms should be close to the rib cage, which the elbows are gently squeezing. The shoulders should be shrugged to initiate the movement of bringing the torso out of the water. Use the core muscles to continue lifting the head and upper torso out of the water at this time, which helps the arms and elbows complete the final inches of the circle (figure 2.12b). As the fingertips approach each other just under the chin and the elbows are beginning to squeeze the ribcage as just noted, still scraping batter off the edge of the bowl, turn the palms inward so that the pinkie sides of the hands meet to form a platform on which to lift the batter to the face (figure 2.12c).

Begin to move the hands forward as the head drops and shoulders relax. The face should come close enough to the hands to lick the batter, keeping elbows squeezed together and palms up. As the hands move past the head and the arms extend away from the body, rotate the palms outward so that by the time the arms are almost at full extension and the hands reenter the water, the body is returning to the modified streamline position (figure 2.12d).

## Kicking

As the fingertips are gathering batter, the bottom half of the legs also complete an arc-like pattern. Unlike the other strokes, in which the toes are pointing back away from the body, the ankles during the breaststroke are at 90-degree angles to the legs at all times unless in the streamline position. The ankle angle is important to the power transfer from the legs to the water.

The kicking motion has three distinct phases: up, out, and together. From the modified streamline position, the knees bend so that the flexed heels come straight toward and almost touch the buttocks. This is the Up phase.

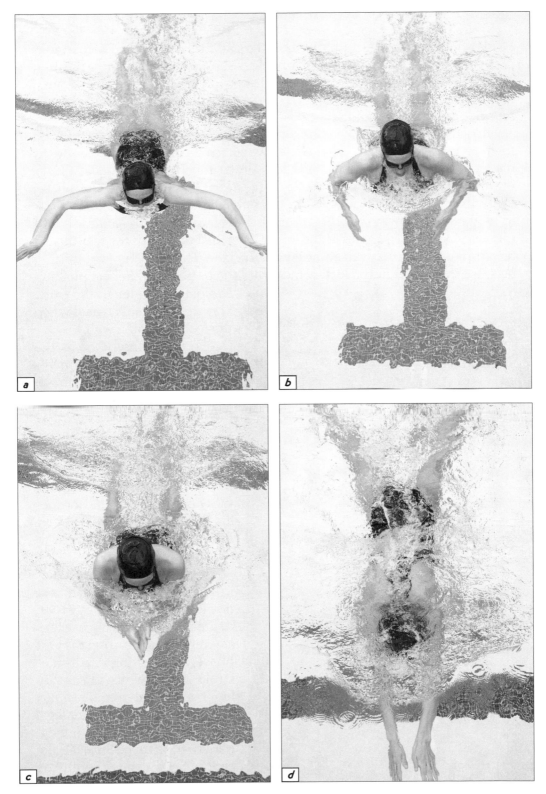

**Figure 2.12** Upper-body movements for the breaststroke: (a) the elbow bend, (b) the inner pull, (c) finishing the pull, and (d) the forward push.

Heels should be in line with the shoulders and turned inward so that toes point to the sides of the pool. The upper legs should be in streamline position with knees close together but not touching; ankles should be at 90-degree angles (figure 2.13a). This position requires good flexibility of the quadriceps muscles and the knee joints.

From the Up position, the knees twist out so that each foot travels through the water in a symmetrical semicircle away from the midline of the body. As the legs rotate in the arc shape, the knees almost touch as they work as a lever in moving the bottom half of the legs (figure 2.13b). This is the Out phase. Done properly, this phase is felt in the outer hip as the hip muscles work to move the feet away from and then back toward the body. Ankles should remain at 90-degree angles to the lower legs; the bottoms of the feet should be parallel to the pool wall at the end of the lane. This imagery is important because the power in the kick comes from the bottoms of the feet pushing against the water in the same way that power is created when the feet push off a wall.

The Out phase ends as the legs straighten and the heels kick into the Together phase, which is back in the streamline position (figure 2.13c). The ankles remain in that 90-degree angle the entire time to maximize the power transfer from the legs through the feet against the water. The only time the toes are pointed away from the body is briefly when they return to the streamline position.

The most common mistakes in the breaststroke kick are not keeping the ankles at 90-degree angles, moving the legs asymmetrically during the Out phase, and drifting into a side-stroke kick in which knees stay together but calves move apart to form a V with the lower legs. If swimmers unfamiliar or inexperienced with the breaststroke choose to try to incorporate the stroke into their training, they should do so gradually. The

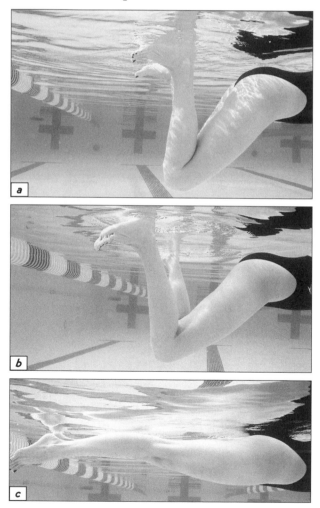

**Figure 2.13** The breaststroke kick: (a) up, (b) out, (c) together.

strain the kick places on the knees could cause knee pain if the muscles in the legs aren't slowly adapted to the motion.

## Timing

Although the movements of the upper body and legs are two separate actions, the timing of these actions is important to maximize power and stay balanced. The movements of the upper body and lower body should start and stop concurrently.

As the hands begin to go out, the feet begin to come up. As the elbows start to bend to accommodate the circumference of the batter bowl, the feet go out. As the hands make their way toward the mouth for the batter to be licked, the feet begin to come together. The final thrust in the water with the legs helps the upper body dive forward toward the streamline position, which the upper body and lower body reach simultaneously. It's as if you kick your hands forward in the Together phase.

## Breathing

The upper-body movement of the breaststroke allows for a natural breathing pattern. As the fingertips trace the last part of the circumference of the bowl and elbows are tight against the rib cage, the lower and middle back muscles contract to arch the back and lift the head and upper body out of the water at a 45-degree angle. The arching of the back is similar to doing a backward half sit-up or a rocking motion. You arch up, and then you rock down. That motion also helps your fingertips trace that last bit of the bowl very close to the body.

Breath is taken from the time the body begins to rise until it reaches its highest position out of the water. Then, when the body is arched back, forearms are touching the rib cage, fingertips have met, and feet are in the Out position, returning to the streamline position is as simple as relaxing the back muscles, kicking the feet together, shooting the hands forward, and placing the head back into the water. The mouth and nose should be exhaling by the time the face and head return to the water, and the face and eyes should end up staring directly at the bottom of the pool.

## Pull-Down

When swimming freestyle or backstroke, the forward momentum in the streamline position after starts and turns is aided by a flutter kick or dolphin kick. The underwater pull-down performs the same function when swimming breaststroke, the only stroke in which the upper body is used in some way other than to maintain streamline position. The hands move to the hips, pushing water to provide more momentum. They then return to streamline position during the kick portion of the pull-down, allowing you to return to the surface of the water. The arm and hand movements provide forward momentum when pushing them toward the hips and as little drag as possible when moving them back to streamline position. This is a different motion than the breaststroke stroke itself.

To begin a pull-down, push off under the water into streamline position. When momentum in the streamline position starts to slow, turn the hands so that fingertips point to the bottom of the pool and palms face the pool wall just kicked off from. Elbows are high and squeezed against the body, as if you're doing an underwater chicken dance. The trapezius muscles between the shoulder blades are flexed, pulling in the shoulders. The hands are then pushed toward the hips very close to the body, following its contour, so that the thumbs almost hit the rib cage. By the time the hands reach the hips and are fully extended, the tops of the hands are facing the bottom of the pool. Fingertips point toward the wall just kicked off from, and shoulders drop, putting the body in a variation of the streamline position. All this time, the legs and feet aren't doing anything. They remain in streamline position.

When momentum fades again, or a breath is needed, the hands return to streamline position as a breaststroke kick torpedoes the body out of the water. To do this, the thumbs begin following the contour of the body as the kick is going through the Up and Out phases. This time, though, the hands remain parallel to the surface of the water to reduce drag. Elbows are kept tight against the body. As the hands move past the chest, palms up, the wrists turn so that fingers form a V by the time they reach the throat and chin. This way they are in position to shoot forward in the normal extension movement of the breaststroke as the Together phase of the kick shoots the body out of the water and back to streamline position.

For competitive breaststrokers, a FINA rule change in 2005 allows for a single downward dolphin kick during a portion of the breaststroke pull-down. Although the details and execution of that rule are outside the scope of this book, the move does increase the forward movement underwater and should be learned if competing is a goal.

# Butterfly

The butterfly might be the hardest of the strokes to learn, but this is not because the movements are difficult. Both the arm motion and the kick are relatively straightforward, but getting the timing down is tricky. In the breaststroke, the upper- and lower-body motions are not movements that come naturally, but choreographing them is clear-cut because they begin and end at the same time. In the butterfly, the actions are simple, but the timing stumps some swimmers. Swimming the butterfly places extra emphasis on the shoulders, core, and hips.

## Upper-Body Movement

As in the breaststroke, both hands work in unison in the butterfly stroke, rather than opposite each other as in the freestyle and backstroke. The early motion of the hands underwater is similar to that of the freestyle stroke, moving in the shape of a backward S. The hands don't leave the water at the hips but continue to push water down the sides of the legs until the arms and hands are fully extended.

The hands enter the water straight in front of the shoulders with fingers spread slightly, thumbs down, and palms facing opposite sides of the pool. From the shoulder-width position, the arms remain straight as the palms move out away from each other and push the water toward the sides of the pool until each arm is about 45 degrees from the midline of the body. The arms themselves are forming a 90-degree angle, with the head splitting the middle. At this point, the elbows bend to allow the palms of the hands to turn and pull water back toward the belly button in a circular arc. Once the thumbs reach the side of the torso in line with the belly button, and the fingertips are pointing to the bottom of the pool, the hands push toward and eventually past the hips, once again in line with the shoulders, until they finally leave the water as far down the legs as the extended arms and hands allow.

Once the hands have left the water, the recovery phase of the stroke begins (figure 2.14a). Just as in freestyle, the goal is to return the hands and arms to the forward position as quickly and naturally as possible (figure 2.14b). The most efficient motion is to keep the thumbs close to the water, almost skimming the top of the pool with the tips of the thumbs. Arms remain extended and straight throughout the recovery, so the path of the hands is in a 180-degree semicircle away from the hips and then back toward and into the streamline position.

Two misconceptions of the butterfly stroke are the position of the hands while beginning the stroke and the movement of the arms during recovery.

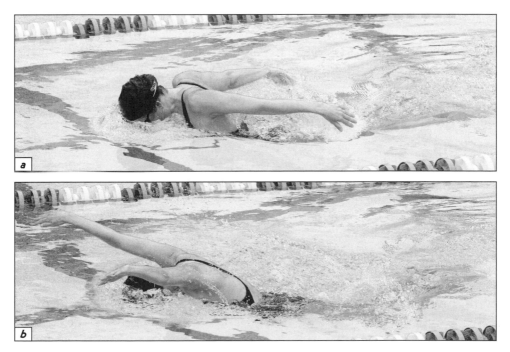

**Figure 2.14** Upper-body recovery in the butterfly stroke.

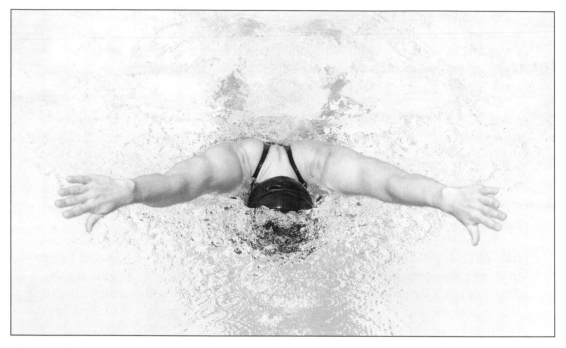

**Figure 2.15** For maximum power in the butterfly stroke, hands should enter the water straight in front of the shoulders.

Many swimmers' hands enter the water touching or very close together, but they should be straight in front of the shoulders (figure 2.15). That position is much stronger than the slight inward angle formed when the hands are close together, which invokes the smaller shoulder muscles rather than the larger, more powerful ones. In the recovery phase of the stroke, a full shoulder revolution that brings the hands far out of the water and above the body and head is unnecessary. This movement increases the distance the hands must travel and thus increases the time before the next stroke can begin (plus it puts added pressure on the shoulder joint).

## Kicking

The butterfly kick is also called the dolphin kick, because the motion somewhat simulates a dolphin swimming in and out of the water. Although in the butterfly stroke, the body doesn't leave the water as the graceful dolphins do, the undulation through the water is the primary image of the butterfly kick.

Just as in the freestyle and backstroke, the kick for the butterfly begins with the hips, not the knees. Similarly, the hamstring muscles should never flex the knee into a 90-degree angle. Although the knees will bend some with the rhythm of the motion of the torso and legs—stiff legs can't properly execute the dolphin kick—those joints should not be used as a source of leverage or power themselves. The real power comes from the lower abdominal muscles working in conjunction with the hips to create the long, continuous, whiplike motion of the entire lower body.

Ankles should be relaxed, and feet should stay together the entire time. In butterfly competition, at no time may the feet execute the dolphin kick separately of each other. Swimmers will be disqualified if the feet ever separate. Keeping the knees close helps the feet remain together and operate as one unit.

The action of the butterfly kick is uncomplicated. The torso and lower body mimic the motion of a dolphin swimming through the water. The wavelike movement starts with the flexing of the abdominal muscles to pull the hips up slightly. By the time the ripple effect causes the legs to raise, the torso and then hips have begun to sink back into the water to lead the downward kick that propels the body.

The natural rhythm of the kick can usually be felt within the first few times of trying the kick in water. The best way to learn the dolphin kick is by using a pair of fins and kicking on the back in streamline position. The exaggerated power the fins generate helps swimmers feel the rhythm of the undulation and the benefit of keeping the feet together, and the supinated position helps swimmers learn the proper position of the knees. An excessive knee bend causes the knees to break the surface of the water, which will be noticeable if swimming on the back.

## Timing

The butterfly kick is slower than the freestyle kick because of the full undulation from the hips through the legs and to the toes. For every stroke there are two kicks: one at the beginning of the stroke and the other at the beginning of the recovery. Thinking about using the kick to aid the arms helps develop the timing and rhythm crucial to an efficient stroke. As hands separate in the early phase of the stroke, the first kick occurs. As hands leave the water and the 180-degree arc begins, the second kick occurs. The cue is to kick hands back and then kick hands forward.

## Breathing

Breathing for the butterfly is as natural as the rest of the stroke. When the arms are fully extended during the final push phase of the stroke, the chin skims along the surface of the water, and a breath is taken. It's not necessary to fully arch the neck to lift the head out of water. Instead, move only enough to accomplish the objective, which in this case is a waterless inhalation. As the hands then begin to come forward, the head returns to streamline position in the water. Breathing every other stroke is recommended.

## Pushoff

A pushoff is used in the butterfly stroke to maximize the distance off the wall after each turn before beginning the stroke and to help rise to the surface of the water. After pushing off the wall in the streamline position, two to three dolphin kicks will get you to the surface. As soon as the hands leave the water, they should be in position to begin the stroke.

If it feels as if you're sinking or staying at the same depth in the water during the pushoff, slightly point the head and hands toward the top of the water. The head and arms control where the body goes in the water, just as a steering wheel controls the direction of a car, and the body will naturally pop to the surface of the water.

# Turns

The various methods swimmers use after pushing off the wall is one example of how swimming technique entails more than simply stroking and kicking from one end of a pool to the other. To varying degrees, starts, turns, and finishes also play central roles in swimming. Obviously, starts and finishes are much more important to swimmers who compete in meets, but all swimmers (aside from those who swim regularly in open water) will need to do dozens, if not hundreds, of turns during every workout. Although learning to perform stroke-specific turns is not vital to improving fitness and conditioning in the pool, swimmers of all goals and abilities can enjoy better continuity in their strokes if they learn the proper turn for each stroke they use. Essentially, there are only two turns in swimming among the four strokes. The turn used in the freestyle and backstroke is almost the same; the only difference is when the swimmer rotates from the back to the belly. There's no difference at all in the turn used for the breaststroke and butterfly.

## Freestyle and Backstroke

The primary element of the turn used when swimming freestyle and backstroke is a half somersault in the water in a tight, tucked position that leaves the feet parallel to the wall with the legs flexed and ready to thrust the body back into streamline position. This technique is also called a *flip turn*.

When swimming freestyle, executing a 180-degree somersault means swimmers will be pushing off from the wall on their backs and must rotate back onto the belly during extension of the legs. When swimming backstroke, swimmers rotate to the stomach before the somersault and are in position to resume the backstroke after pushing away from the wall. First I'll describe executing the turn when swimming freestyle; I'll follow with the variations used when swimming backstroke.

The turn in freestyle begins when one hand is at the hip and the other hand is about to enter the water. Push the chin to the clavicle very tightly, as if trying to fit the chin into the indention of the collarbone just below the throat (figure 2.16a). The two body parts seem to be made for this very purpose. Bring the knees to the chest and the hand that is just about to enter the water to the hip so that the body is in as tight a tuck as possible, almost in a fetal position. Do a forward roll until the back is facing the bottom of the pool (figure 2.16b). The bottom of the feet should be parallel to the pool wall, with toes pointing straight up toward the ceiling or sky; knees should form a 90-degree angle. Essentially, the movement is similar to doing a half somersault right before the wall.

From that tight tuck, plant the feet solidly on the wall (figure 2.16c) and push off as hard as you can on your back. Imagine the body as a coil springing from the wall. During the pushoff (figure 2.16d), the hands begin extending forward as the body rotates like a corkscrew 180 degrees to return to the freestyle position with belly facing the pool bottom (figure 2.16e). The turn can be made either clockwise or counterclockwise, whichever is more comfortable, and the result is the streamline position. Because all of this is happening underwater, a dolphin kick or freestyle kick helps propel the body both forward and upward to the surface in preparation for the first stroke.

Two common mistakes are made when executing the flip turn, and they are interrelated. Some swimmers are lazy and throw their legs over their bodies instead of tucking into compact balls. The result leads to the second problem, which is not being in

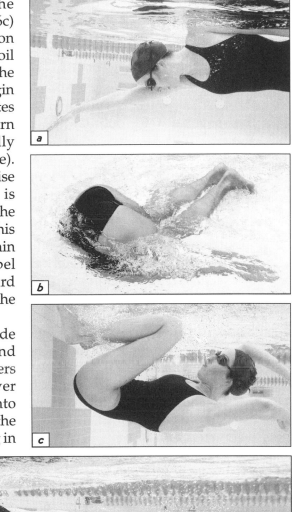

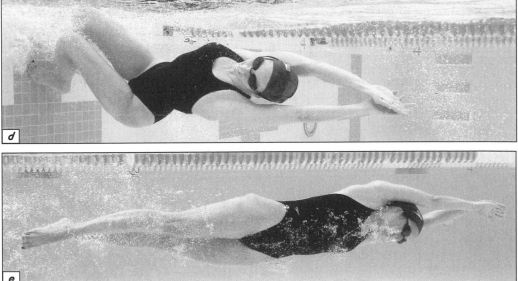

**Figure 2.16** The freestyle flip turn: (a) pushing chin to clavicle, (b) beginning the forward roll, (c) planting feet on the wall, (d) the pushoff, and (e) returning to the freestyle position.

position to plant the feet on the wall with knees at 90-degree angles. If the toes barely reach the wall or the legs are only slightly bent, the potential energy in that coiled spring is wasted and velocity off the wall is minimal.

Knowing when to begin the flip turn is a matter of personal preference and comfort. It takes time to master the delicate blend of five elements: the distance away from the wall at which the swimmer's final stroke concludes, the speed at which the swimmer is traveling, the distance it takes to execute the somersault, the optimal distance away from the wall each individual should be before planting the feet, and the aggressiveness of the swimmer. Aggressive swimmers will want to turn as close to the wall as possible to achieve a tighter coil. Some swimmers are concerned about hitting their heels on the gutters and so turn farther away from the wall.

The good news is that virtually every pool has lane lines that form a T at the end of the lane and a marker on the wall to help cue when the turn should begin. The end of the T on the bottom of the pool should not signal that the turn begins immediately but rather how many more strokes should be executed before beginning the somersault. This number of strokes differs among swimmers depending on their stroke length, stroke efficiency, and willingness to turn close to the wall. One way to find the perfect place to begin the turn is to experiment when not swimming laps. Find a somewhat open place about three to five feet (1-1.5 meters) from the pool wall, noting how far you are from the edge. Do a full somersault in the water and land on your feet. Then compare the distance from where you started to where you finished. That distance plus the length of your torso in the coiled position should be about the distance from the wall at which your flip should begin.

The turn when swimming backstroke begins with the swimmer rotating onto the belly for one freestyle stroke to move him or her into position to begin the flip turn, whereas in the freestyle, the corkscrew motion takes place after the flip turn. In competition, only one freestyle stroke right before the wall on a backstroke turn is allowed. If more than one freestyle stroke is taken, the swimmer is disqualified.

The direction of the backstroke rotation depends on which arm begins the stroke, and this choice is intuitive and natural. If the right hand is entering the water, the rotation is clockwise from the back to the belly, and the left hand becomes closest to the approaching wall by the time the rotation is complete. If the left hand is entering the water, the rotation is counterclockwise onto the belly, and the right hand becomes the closest to the approaching wall by the time the rotation is complete. After the spring off the wall on the back, the hands move forward until the arms are extended and the body has returned to the streamline position. Then a few butterfly or backstroke kicks propel the body to the surface of the water.

When swimming the backstroke, look for the flags hanging above the pool; these are the cue to when the turn should begin to take place. Most

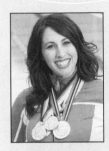

## Flip Turns

Learning to flip turn for freestyle and backstroke can be a little daunting for adults who have not grown up swimming on club teams. I was about four when I learned the flip turn, so I don't remember much about the learning process. Executing the half somersault is only part of the battle—you also need to perfect the timing of the initiation of the flip.

Getting that timing down is fully personal preference. Most average-sized people will take two normal strokes after the T. You might find that taking two stretched-out strokes or three shortened strokes works better for you. To give you some perspective, I take just one freestyle stroke after I see the T before starting the flip. In backstroke, after I see the flag, I take two strokes, rotating to my belly on the second, and take one freestyle stroke before starting the flip.

beginners take about three or four strokes after passing under the flags before spiraling onto their bellies.

The final but extremely important point to remember when executing a flip turn is to continue blowing air out of the nose. As discussed earlier, it's very difficult to keep water out of the nose when air is not leaving the nostrils. When some swimmers first learn the flip turn, they get caught up in the body movements and forget to continuously expel water from the nose.

## Breaststroke and Butterfly

The turn executed when swimming the breaststroke or butterfly begins with both hands touching the wall at the same time, which is mandatory in any official race. If the swimmer were to be frozen in time at the instant the turn begins, the hands would be planted firmly on the wall shoulder-width apart at the ends of outstretched arms, and the body would be in streamline position.

But the swimmer is not frozen in time. Instead, with both hands on the wall, she uses her momentum to begin bringing her knees to her chest. Beginners might even grab the edge of the gutter to help pull themselves to the wall. Once both hands are on the wall, one arm quickly leaves the wall and begins to move in a backward motion led by the elbow (figure 2.17a).

As the elbow continues to move toward the opposite end of the pool, the knees continue to bend toward the chest in an effort to plant both feet on the wall (figure 2.17b). Just before the feet hit the wall, the head is raised for a breath and the backward moving arm begins to move in a 180-degree clockwise or counterclockwise motion under the surface of the water (figure 2.17c).

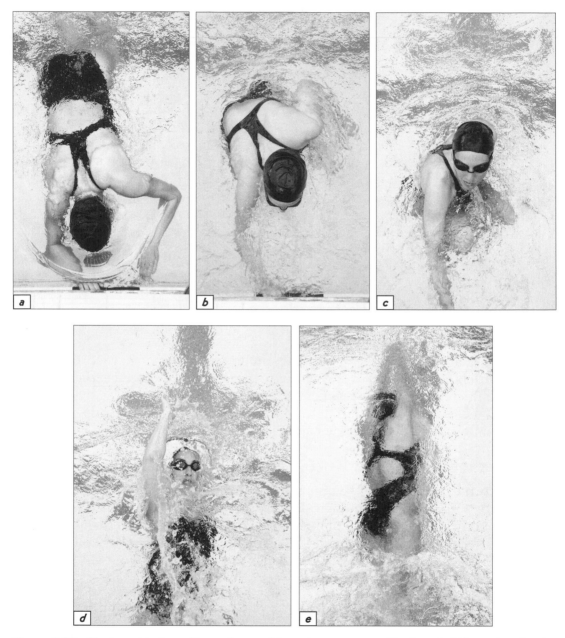

**Figure 2.17** The breaststroke and butterfly turn: *(a)* arm begins to extend backward, *(b)* knees bend to the chest, *(c)* head raises and hand moves in a 180-degree motion, *(d)* the karate chop, and *(e)* the pushoff.

After the feet are planted, the opposite hand executes a karate chop next to the corresponding ear, and the pushoff begins (figure 2.17d). The feet twist on the wall, and the body twists in the direction of the hand moving under the water; so, at one brief point during the spring off the wall, the swimmer is actually on one side and quickly moving to the belly. Legs thrust off the wall as the hand that has been by the ear moves forward to meet the other arm at the top of the head, and the arms and body assume the streamline position (figure 2.17e).

Executing the turn for the breaststroke and butterfly is not as difficult as the flip turn, nor is it as important to maintaining a rhythm in the pool. Because it is similar to simply reaching the wall and changing direction, fitness swimmers would be better served concentrating on improving their actual strokes than on improving this turn. However, competitors will want to practice bringing the knees tight to the chest to make the turn as efficient as possible, instead of wasting energy turning an elongated body through the water.

# chapter 3

# Swim Training Guidelines

Just as you can't jump into the water and know how to swim well the first time you try, swim training also takes some getting used to. To the uninitiated, the basic phrases and concepts common in swim training are foreign and meaningless. Even those who have been swimming laps for years might find some of the workout jargon unfamiliar or not understand precisely how improvement in the pool occurs. The guidelines in this chapter lay the foundation for beginning the workouts in part II and using the programs in part III. Through these workouts and programs, you will be able to meet your goals as a swimmer. This chapter will look at the steps through which swim fitness is built, including the all-important habit of charting your progress. It will also discuss the typical segments of a standard swim workout, the concept of interval training, and methods of gauging your effort in the pool. Finally, I'll review some tips on how to avoid injuries and prevent tweaks from developing into full-blown problems.

## Building Swim Fitness

Swimming is an unnatural activity in the sense that people do very little, if anything, to replicate it outside of the pool. Walking is an everyday activity, and everyone has run somewhere, whether it's across the yard, the neighborhood, or the city. Picking up objects of various degrees of heaviness and in different ways is common, as is bending over, kneeling down, squatting, pushing, pulling, holding, twisting, lugging, hauling, and balancing. But the movements of the arms, torso, and legs when swimming the freestyle, backstroke, breaststroke, or butterfly rarely or never happen outside of swim training. That ultimately is good news because improvement will come relatively quickly for those who swim regularly. Initially, though, it might feel like the opposite is true; the act of merely getting from one end of the pool to the other might feel impossible the first time you try. The unique muscle movements of swimming create a steep learning curve, and both new and experienced swimmers will see progress more quickly by focusing on the five phases of improvement in the optimal order. If swimmers apply these concepts to their workouts and continually challenge themselves, they'll see significant results. The results don't come overnight, however. Setting goals and charting your progress in a log book is extremely motivating because you can look back over the weeks and months of workouts and marvel at how far you have come.

## Five Steps to Success

Improving as a swimmer is a five-step process, and all but the most elite swimmers can see significant gains in their fitness levels and performances in each of the phases. The first and most important stage is learning to breathe, and this is followed closely by the second most important: getting comfortable in the water. The two are closely related because it's hard to be relaxed if you can't breathe. Learning to blow bubbles (using the exercise in chapter 2) and to float on your back are two ways to ease the tension of being in the water.

At the third stage, the focus is on flexing the core muscles and honing stroke technique. Early in this stage, swimmers must consciously engage the abdominal, hip, and lower back muscles, concentrating on the feeling of using them to keep the body in the streamline position. Having excellent form in each stroke isn't a prerequisite for getting exercise in the pool; even people who flail from one end of the pool to the other can get a fine workout. But they won't be able to improve much because of the vast amount of energy it takes them merely to move through the water.

Following stroke mechanics, the fourth stage is to build a fitness base in the water. Fitness on land does not equate to fitness in the water. Effort in water is greater than effort on land, and swimmers must appreciate that. Newer or returning swimmers should start out swimming 1 to 4 laps at a time, resting after each group, and shoot to cover 10 to 20 laps in the first couple of workouts. They should do as much as they can without making the experience negative to the point that they don't want to return. They should then add 1 to 4 laps to each successive workout and gradually decrease the rest they take until they can swim 30 or 40 laps with minimal rest.

The fifth and final stage of development is working on turns and increasing intensity and total distance in workouts. Swimming dozens of straight laps is very good exercise, and fitness will improve up to a point. But eventually progress will plateau because the body's muscular and cardiovascular systems are no longer being taxed in ways different enough to produce marked improvement. The body is wonderfully adaptive to almost anything we throw at it. If we decide to take a new route to work, at first that route will be unfamiliar and require more thought than the old route. But soon the mind and body become accustomed to the thousands of new stimuli and movements necessary to go that route, and driving it becomes second nature. The same goes for training. A new workout regimen is difficult at first. Muscles break down. The body gets sore. Fatigue sets in. Pretty quickly, though, the body figures out that some physiological changes will make things easier. As great as that might sound, eventually progress will plateau. The physiological principle that aided improvement in the first place—the body's ability to adapt—ultimately can lead to a downfall. Once the body becomes fully adjusted to a particular workout or type of training, it has no further incentive to change, and the rate of improvement dwindles.

All athletes must fully understand and appreciate, emotionally as well as mentally, that physical progress is an ongoing process. You don't check off step 1 after you can breathe in the water and then rush through the other four steps to magically become an elite swimmer. Instead, with progress, the focus of each facet of improvement changes. After getting comfortable with breathing, attention turns to improving lung capacity. Getting comfortable in the water is replaced with developing a feel for the water with the hands and forearms. Stroke mechanics progress from honing gross motor skills of the hands, arms, legs, and core to the finer points of slight angle changes and other minute details that lower times and improve fitness.

## Setting Goals

We have all heard about the importance of setting goals in various aspects of life. Deciding what you want to accomplish and mapping out a plan for what needs to be done is important to staying on track for any endeavor. I was a very good swimmer as a child, but only after I truly set goals and knew what it would take to accomplish them did my swimming career really take off. Everyone's goals will be different. What is common to goals is that setting them nearly always helps create focus and produce results. To be most effective, goals must be specific and challenging but also realistic. Those three elements—specific, challenging, realistic—are what makes a goal motivating. For instance, a new fitness swimmer's goal to keep up in the fast lane at a masters workout within a month is unrealistic. The goal itself—being a fast member of a masters team—is excellent, but the deadline will surely bring disappointment.

When people think of goals, they often focus on the long term or end result: lowering a time, winning a race, losing inches off the waist, keeping up in the fast lane. Some goals, though, are process oriented, such as improving a particular aspect of a stroke, learning a flip turn, or swimming a certain number of days or a particular distance a week. These goals are still specific and can be valuable either on their own or as stepping-stones

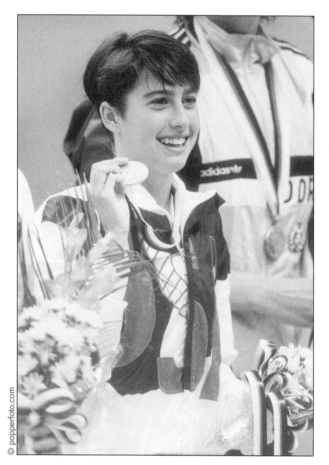

© popperfoto.com

Working hard toward my goals paid off when I beat the East Germans in the 400-meter freestyle at the 1988 Olympics.

to achieve an ultimate goal. The swimmer who sets a series of short-term goals in line with the process of improving will be more successful than the one who sets long-term goals with no real plan for getting there. For example, first working on technique and then swimming a certain number of laps in one workout before introducing intervals into training and, finally, lowering those intervals to achieve a desired result is a great way to use smaller goals as steps toward achieving larger ones.

## Charting Your Progress

Many swimmers find it motivating to keep a log book. There is no better way to witness the progress being made than by writing down every aspect of each of your workouts. Although improvement happens daily, it's often hard to recognize it without stepping back a bit. The saying "You can't see the forest for the trees" applies here. Overall progress can be hard to detect when your daily focus is on individual workouts. But when discouragement sets in or time is not falling off in chunks, it can be uplifting to look back through previous workouts to see the progress you have made.

The sooner you begin recording your workouts, the better. The first thing new swimmers should do is buy a notebook and chronicle their workouts from the start, but swimmers of any level and ability, including the most advanced, will benefit from charting the details of each session in the pool. The information recorded in the log books can be quite straightforward and general, extremely detailed, or somewhere in between, depending on individual preference. At the very least you should write down every component of the day's training, including your swim workout (sets, distances, and times); any nonswimming workout (the type, distance, time, weight routine, etc.); time spent stretching; and any core work (the number and type of exercises). Here is an example of a simple log entry:

### Simple Workout Log

| | |
|---|---|
| Preswim workout: | 30 min on bike at 12 mph, 15 min on treadmill at 3.0 mph and 5.0 grade |
| Stretching: | 12 min |
| Sit-ups: | 5 × 50 of normal sequence |
| Swimming: | 200 free warm-up |
| | 25 laps with 20-sec rest between 50s and 2-min rest between sets of 5 |
| | 150 free cool-down |

For some swimmers, a simple log book is sufficient, whereas others like to go into much more detail. In general, the more information that's recorded, the easier it is to analyze past workouts and current progress. For some, the time it takes to remember and write down the details is not worth the effort. Their goals are more process oriented than outcome oriented, and studying which weeks were good and which were not is not important to them. For others, though, especially competitors, knowing how they felt during a particular workout or noticing a pattern of especially good or bad workouts can be extremely helpful in preparing for the next race or season. In fact, log books usually aren't optional when you swim on a team, and they become more necessary as the competition gets better. The usefulness of a log book is not restricted to swimmers. Coaches also use log books frequently, studying how an athlete performed in past workouts before writing future workouts. Details of interval, total distance, times, and athlete comments about workouts are invaluable in planning for the next season. For those groups, and for those who find statistics and details fascinating, a more detailed log is advantageous. Here's an example:

### Detailed Workout Log

| | |
|---|---|
| Preswim workout: | 15 min on bike at 10 mph—ES 3 |
| | 30 min on treadmill at 3.5 mph and 5.0 grade—ES 6 |
| Stretching: | 12 min—felt especially tight today |
| Sit-ups: | 5 × 25 normal sequence—these are getting easier; go up to 30 tomorrow |
| Swimming: | 2,500 yards / 60 min—overall pretty good day; yardage getting easier |
|    Warm-up: | 300 free |
|    Kick set: | 8 × 25 on 1:00 (no fins) with 50 swim down—still tough to get through |
|    Pull set: | 4 × 75 on 1:45 (buoy/paddles)—feel good progress on pulling |
|    Main set: | 1 × 25 on :30, 1 × 50 on 1:00, 1 × 75 on 1:30, 1 × 100 on 2:00 |
| | Repeat 4 times—held 26-27 sec/25 on all but 3rd, and 4th 100 was 28-29 sec/25 |

| | |
|---|---|
| Sprint set: | 4 × 50 on 1:30—didn't feel fast today; went 42 sec, 44 sec, 43 sec, 46 sec |
| Drill set: | 1 × 50 H-S-F, 1 × 50 free, 1 × 50 FLA r/l, 1 × 50 free, 1 × 50 Fr 3-3-3 |
| Cool-down: | 200 switching between free and back per 25 |

I can't emphasize enough how important it is to keep a log book. It might seem hard enough to remember a workout at the pool, much less the times for each lap, and it might be next to impossible at first. With experience, paying attention to details becomes second nature, and each week more and more details stick with you. Recording the workout while still at the pool will help you get the details down before they're pushed out of your mind by other facts and information. The process itself is therapeutic and motivating. Inspiration comes not only from flipping back through the pages to see how much faster you now swim or how substantial the gradual increase in total distance has become but also from simply wanting to record a positive workout.

I encourage swimmers to gain an appreciation for the rate at which progress takes place. A lack of understanding can bring frustration and dejection if expectations are unreasonable. Frustration and dejection too often are followed by skipping workouts here and there or quitting the sport altogether, so avoiding the mistake of expecting too much too soon will do wonders for your improvement in your swimming and fitness level. There's no infomercial claiming that swimming guarantees the loss of 10 pounds in 10 days or your money back. Results come gradually, and what results you get depends heavily on how long you've been swimming, how frequently you swim, and how hard you work in the pool.

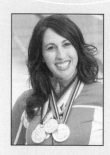

# Legendary Log Books

As I have mentioned, log books can be inspirational for athletes in seeing how far they have come. It can also be inspirational for coaches to view log books of athletes from other teams. Coming up with different ways to write workouts that are both effective and engaging can get challenging, and looking over different log books can jump-start a coach's creative juices.

In the swimming world, my log books reached urban legend status. The amount of training I put in and the pace at which I swam my workouts were crazy. My 1988 log book especially was passed around from coach to coach, who found new ways to challenge their teams. Swimmers would dread their coach getting his or her hands on my log book because they knew they'd have an especially tough workout in the near future!

Swimming can be frustrating. The unique set of movements and skills involved in swimming are not mastered overnight. Remembering that reality helps. There will be days when your stroke feels great and muscle memory seems to have taken over, and then the next day you're thrashing through the water as if you've never been wet. Expect to be discouraged occasionally. The body goes through stages during which strength and endurance gains seem to occur rapidly; other times, progress might stall. Start slowly. To get a sense of your current fitness level, take the maximum heart rate swim test that appears later in the chapter. Don't try to add more than several laps to any one workout if you're just beginning; don't add more than a few hundred yards at a time if you're advanced. Allow muscles in the body to learn the technique, to break down during the workout, and to build themselves back up in time for the next one.

# Anatomy of a Workout

I hope you now appreciate the importance of building and tracking your swim fitness, if you didn't already. Now let's move to discussing the structure of a swim workout and the role various components play in the development of a swimmer. Not all workouts are the same, of course, but most are divided into different sections called sets. Several types of sets can be found in the workouts in this book, although all sets will not appear in all workouts. Each set contains at least two repetitions, or reps, of a particular distance. For instance, if a workout calls for swimming 100 yards 10 times (written 10 × 100), each 100 yards is considered a rep. Technically there's no limit to the number of reps in a set. The recommended percentage of the day's total distance that each set should comprise is approximate and will fluctuate somewhat because the recommendation assumes that all sets are included in every workout. The order of the sets is also somewhat flexible, except that each workout should always begin with a warm-up and conclude with a cool-down.

## Warm-Up

The warm-up is an important part of every workout because it prepares all the muscles that will be used in swimming to fully exert themselves. About 10 to 20 percent of the length of the workout should be swum at an easy pace that requires minimal effort; the exertion should be similar to that of a slow walk. The strokes should be very long, and the focus should be on stretching out the upper body and getting the blood flowing before asking the heart to start pumping hard in subsequent sets.

Tune in to your body to get a read on how you feel in the water each day. Some days you might feel fast, other days steady, and some days sluggish, just like in life. Getting a sense of how you feel helps you prepare mentally for the most challenging segments of a workout. If you're feeling tense or apprehensive, no matter the cause, try blowing bubbles underwater to help you relax. Make sure your gear is easily accessible and organized at the side of the pool. Stop to adjust your cap or goggles if necessary so you don't have to interrupt the meat of the workout and lose even the slightest chance to improve fitness that day.

If a workout includes more than the freestyle, you'll want to warm up the other strokes you'll be swimming that day. It's best not to warm up the butterfly until you're fully warmed up in the other strokes because even at warm-up pace, the butterfly stroke is more strenuous than the others. Simple butterfly drills will suffice instead of swimming the full stroke during the warm-up. Toward the end of the warm-up, effort should increase slightly to ensure muscles are loose and ready for the more strenuous sets to come.

Even when pinched for time, it's best not to skip the warm-up. Doing so invites injury by forcing the body to work hard before it's ready and also decreases the effectiveness of your swimming effort. The body simply doesn't perform at peak levels unless it has had a chance to warm up in the specific way that you'll be working out. This means the additional "quality" laps you think you're getting by skipping the warm-up aren't so quality after all.

## Drill Set

About 5 to 7 percent of your total distance should be spent drilling. All swimmers—from the beginner to the world-record holder—should incorporate drills into their regular training regimens. My last workout at my last Olympics included a drill set. Every drill is designed to reinforce one or more aspects of a stroke so that proper form becomes an ingrained motor behavior. If technique is not continually fine-tuned through drills that develop good habits, it will begin to deteriorate and bad habits will be reinforced. Chapter 4 contains 20 stroke-specific drills to aid you in your quest for perfect strokes. As you do for the warm-up, drill for each stroke to be swum that day.

## Kick Set

Another 10 percent of a workout's total distance should be spent kicking. Virtually all kick sets are best done with a kickboard, and some also call for the use of fins. Infrequently, the drill set and kick set will be combined. Again, the kick set should include kicking all strokes to be swum during a session, with focus on technique. An important follow-up to the kick set is the swim down. Holding the arms in a static position on a kickboard for several laps often makes them tighten up. Swimming an easy 100 yards or so will loosen them up again.

## Pull Set

The pull set should be about 20 percent of your workout and is best done with the use of a pull buoy and paddles. The pull set works the shoulders and allows you to focus on upper-body technique. A variation of the pull set is a paddles and fins set, in which the equipment used is modified from the standard pull buoys and paddles to paddles and fins.

# A Day at the Pool for an Olympic Medalist Hopeful

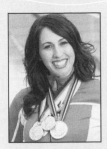

As a 12-year-old, attending the opening ceremonies and swimming competition at the 1984 Olympic Games in Los Angeles was beyond inspiring for me. I had competed since I was five but mostly for fun. Watching the pomp and circumstance of the athletes parading into the stadium behind their countries' flags, followed later by the thrill of the medal ceremonies, lighted a competitive fire and desire in me that could not be extinguished.

I began training seriously with the goal of becoming an Olympian and swimming in the 1988 Games in Seoul, South Korea. My daily distance increased gradually until I was swimming between 15,000 and 18,000 meters a day spread over two workouts, and I qualified for the Olympics in the 400-meter freestyle, 800-meter freestyle, and 400-meter IM. Less than two months before my first medal ceremony after winning the 400 IM, I swam the following double workout:

| **Tuesday, June 28, 1988** | **16,500 meters** |
|---|---|

| **5:30 — 8:00 a.m.** | **9,000 meters** |
|---|---|
| Warm-up | 500 meters |
| Main set | 8,000 meters |
| 20 × 400 IM | |
|    #s 1-4 on 6:00 | |
|    #s 5-8 on 5:50 | |
|    #s 9-12 on 5:40 | |
|    #s 13-16 on 5:30 (actual times swum—5:19, 5:16, 5:15, 5:15) | |
|    #s 17-20 on 5:20 (actual times swum—5:12, 5:09, 5:07, 5:04) | |
| Cool-down | 500 meters |

| **4:30 — 6:30 p.m.** | **7,500 meters** |
|---|---|
| Warm-up | 800 meters |
| Main set | 6,100 meters |
| 14 × 150 freestyle | |
|    #1 easy on 2:05 | |
|    #2 fast on 1:45 | |
|    #3 easy on 2:05 | |
|    #s 4-5 fast on 1:45 | |
|    #6 easy on 2:05 | |
|    #s 7-9 fast on 1:45 | |
|    #10 easy on 2:05 | |
|    #s 11-14 fast on 1:45 | |

*(continued)*

*(continued)*

Ladder set
4 × 50 easy freestyle on :45
1 × 200 fast backstroke on 2:45
1 × 200 fast breaststroke on 3:00
3 × 100 easy freestyle on 1:25
1 × 150 fast backstroke on 2:05
1 × 150 fast breaststroke on 2:15
2 × 150 easy freestyle on 2:05
1 × 100 fast backstroke on 1:20
1 × 100 fast breaststroke on 1:30
1 × 200 easy freestyle on 2:45
1 × 50 fast backstroke on :45 (actual time swum—:32.8)
1 × 50 fast breaststroke on :45 (actual time swum—:38.1)
*Repeat ladder set 2 times*
Pull set                                                                  600 meters
600 meters freestyle

This day of training was one of my most difficult of the season. My morning workout was obviously the hardest—20 × 400 IMs are very challenging. I was always proud of this particular workout, because even though the main set was 8,000 meters, my last few 400 IMs were swum at a very fast pace. At the 1988 Olympics, I won the 400 IM in a 4:37, and in the above practice, I swam a 5:04 on the last repeat of the set. Training this fast in the workout definitely helped me swim fast at the Olympics!

## Main Set

The main set represents about 35 to 45 percent of the workout and, as the name implies, is the heart of the workout. The success or measure of a workout session usually lies in how well the main set is swum or how the swimmer feels during the set. The makeup of the main set will vary depending on the nature of training for a given day. An endurance set might call for 3 × 500; a speed set might require swimming 20 × 50 as fast as possible but with more rest than usual.

## Speed Set

Regardless of whether the focus of the main set is sprinting, a shorter speed set should comprise about 5 to 10 percent of the workout. Speed sets allow swimmers to maintain the power they have built. At certain times of the season, power will be more of a focus during workouts, but always try to add that bit of sprinting to every workout to stay sharp.

## Cool-Down

Just as important as preparing the body to work hard before a workout is allowing the heart rate to slow down gradually and the shoulders to stretch out after a workout. Both a proper warm-up and cool-down are necessary to make your next workout easier. If you get out of the pool without cooling down, your blood, still coursing rapidly through your vessels, begins to slow down rapidly and settle unevenly, which makes your whole body tighten up. You won't feel the postworkout benefits to the degree that you should, and you'll feel worse than you should the next day in the pool as well. Ending a workout without cooling down is like running a racehorse in the Kentucky Derby and not walking it afterward.

The cool-down should be about the same distance or just a little less than the warm-up, about 10 percent of the total distance for the day. The cool-down should be the easiest set of the day. In the warm-up, maximum effort should equate to a slow walk; in the cool-down, maximum effort should equate to a saunter, or a very slow walk.

Some swimmers tend to neglect the cool-down for a couple of reasons. They are tired and just want to get out of the pool, or they might start thinking about other appointments or errands and feel stressed about fitting everything in. What some don't realize is how hard they've worked their bodies during a good swim workout. It can be more motivating to do the cool-down in sets. On days when you just can't see yourself staying in the pool for an easy, short distance like 400 yards, break it up into 4 × 100 at a very easy interval, or swim part of the cool-down using the backstroke or breaststroke to add variety. Do whatever it takes to stay in the pool long enough to allow the heart rate to slow down.

# Interval Training

Once you have a feel for the different phases of a workout and their purposes, it's time to begin applying the principle of interval training. Every workout in part II—and in fact every swim workout that's not a simple swim—is designed using either rest intervals or base intervals. Interval-based workouts help combat the body's ability to adapt to workouts and the mind's tendency to wander off or get bored during workouts.

The definition of an interval is a pause between two events. In the case of swim training, the pause is between a set number of laps. Rather than swimming the entire distance of a workout with no rest, in an interval-based workout you break up the total distance into preestablished chunks. Let's use a 1,000-yard workout as an example. There are endless ways to swim the laps other than all at once. One is swimming 10 × 100. Even within that configuration, there are two ways to structure the workout. One is to allow a certain amount of rest between each 100, regardless of how fast they are swum. This method is called a rest interval and is the basis of the workouts in chapter 5.

The other method is to begin each 100 at a certain time, leaving equal gaps between each start. You may decide to push off from the wall every

2:00 to swim 100 yards. The amount of rest is based directly on the speed at which you swim those 100 yards. If you swim them in 1:30, you get to rest 30 seconds. If you swim them in 1:50, your break is cut to 10 seconds. The motivation for swimming faster is heightened by the prospect of a longer breather between each 100; this often leads to better gains than a rest interval, which offers no real incentive to push yourself. This type of interval, which is the basis for all workouts except for those in chapter 5, is called a base interval.

The way in which the total distance is broken up and the pace at which it is swum is part of what gives swim workouts variety and stimulates the body's muscles to develop more consistently. Interval training is motivating because it both establishes a benchmark for progress and generates progress.

## Using a Pace Clock

To properly follow an interval-based workout, you need to know how to read and use a pace clock. The basics are easy enough, but a less-obvious use can prove increasingly helpful as workouts get longer. Many if not most pools have at least one pace clock on the pool deck or wall. Swimmers use these timepieces during swimming workouts to time laps, structure interval training, and regulate rest between laps or sets. Use of a pace clock or digital watch is necessary to properly execute almost all of the workouts in this book.

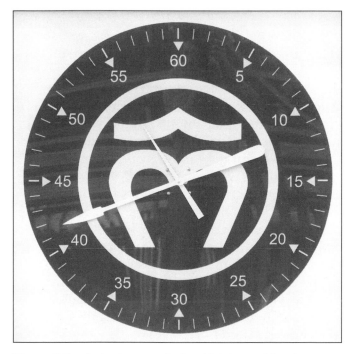

**Figure 3.1**  A classic pace clock, which is considered a necessity for a successful interval-based swim workout.

Although some pace clocks are digital, most are large-face clocks with numbers positioned as on a regular clock. Usually there is only one hand on a pace clock, a second hand, so each number represents 5 seconds that have elapsed in any given minute (figure 3.1). If hash-marks appear between the numbers, they each represent 1 second. When the hand is in the 1 o'clock position, 5 seconds have elapsed in that minute. (In swimming lingo, the hand is said to be "on the 5.") When the hand is at the 2 o'clock position, 10 seconds have elapsed.

The 12 o'clock position, or "60," is called "the top," and 6 o'clock, or "30," is called "the bottom."

A pace clock is the official timepiece of a workout and should be an integral part of all swim training that has improved fitness and performance as objectives. Serious swimmers sometimes hate the clock and feel certain the hand moves more quickly than it should. Some days they might consider "tripping" over the power cord to put the clock out of action. Some nights they will dream of cutting the cord in half. But if you want to improve, the pace clock can be your best friend. Its large face and steady hand are there to keep you on track for each lap, set, and workout. The clock keeps you from lingering too long at the wall when you might otherwise fall behind to take a few more deep breaths. The clock also motivates you to push through a rep so that you actually earn those extra breaths at the wall. Your reward for using a pace clock properly and steadfastly is huge strides in progress.

Pace clocks with a face can provide another function during swim workouts: keeping track of where you are in a set. Suppose your workout calls for swimming 6 × 50 on 1:10. For the first 50, you leave at the top. For the second, you leave at the 10, because that's 1:10 after you left for the first. For the third, you leave at the 20, and so forth. If you stay on pace, literally counting laps isn't necessary because you know you'll leave at the 50 on the last one. Knowing where the hand should be when you push off for each interval is a handy skill to acquire. It's not quite as important for a 300-yard set as it is in a 3,000-yard set, but it's good to learn to think that way from the beginning so you're ready for the longer sets when they come. Often the hardest part is remembering where the hand was when you started the set, so pushing off at the top (12 o'clock) or bottom (6 o'clock) is recommended.

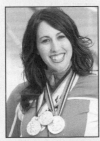

# Outclocked by the Coach

Swim practices for elite distance athletes are grueling, as you might expect, with total daily distances reaching into double-digit miles. Consequently, the sets within those workouts are extremely long, and the rest built into each interval is undoubtedly shorter than we'd prefer.

On days when the main set seemed almost impossible—whether because of the distance, the base, or energy level—my teammates and I would try to skip a few hundred yards by "miscounting" the repeats. Say the main set called for 10 × 200. We'd stop at eight and claim to be finished. We didn't do this at every workout, of course, or even at very many of them. Somehow, though, our coach always knew when to check our work, and he'd do it by reading the clock. He'd know where the hand should be for each 200, and if the hand wasn't where it was supposed to be when we finished, he'd point us back to the pool.

# Calculating Your Base

In base interval workouts, the "base" is the amount of time between each lap or set of laps. Knowing how to calculate and adjust your base helps you tailor workouts to your ability level and make steady improvement in the pool. Each swimmer's base should be established on a swim of 50 yards and then adjusted to the actual distance to be swum. A reasonable base for 50 yards is 1:00 (one minute), so to establish your base, divide the total distance to be swum by 50, and then multiply that number by 1:00. Written out, the formula looks like this:

$$\left(\frac{\text{total distance to be swum}}{50}\right) \times 1:00$$

For a 100, you would divide 100 by 50 and multiply that number by 1:00, resulting in a 100 base of 2:00. The 25 base would be 30 seconds, the 200 base would be 4:00, and so on. (Base conversions for metric pools can be found in the part II opener.)

An important factor in using base interval training to improve is the speed at which each repetition is swum. Holding a pace, or swimming each rep at a consistent speed, should be the goal for fitness swimmers. In a set of 10 × 50 on 1:00 (commonly spoken as "swimming 10 50s on a minute"), it's easy to swim a faster pace on the first few 50s before fatigue sets in. Maybe you were feeling good the first three or four and swam the 50s in 45 seconds, meaning you were holding 45s. But then your shoulders started to tire, your breathing became more difficult, and you swam the next couple in 47 seconds, then 49, then 52, and so on. Learning to swim at the same pace throughout a set enables you to improve at a faster rate than starting out fast and tailing off, even if you're able to make the base time on each repetition.

The way to raise fitness levels and lower times is to strive to lower the base. After several weeks of consistent, challenging workouts, swimming 10 × 50 on 1:00 gets easier. You may go from holding 55s to holding 50s to holding 45s. You're getting comfortable in the water, you're comfortable with the distance and pace, and you start to coast a bit. Now is the time to lower your base.

The amount of rest allowed between repeats is built into the base, but there's such a thing as too much rest. The point of the rest between repeats isn't to allow your heart rate to return to normal. In fact, the converse is true. Rest should be kept to a minimum during most sets so that the heart rate stays somewhat consistent, which leads more quickly to improved fitness. The short break is a chance to take a deep breath, look at the clock, check to see what times you're holding, quickly collect yourself, and push off again. If you find yourself really cruising through a long endurance set with more than 10 seconds of rest between reps, challenge yourself by lowering your base 5 seconds per 100 or 200.

The amount of rest to be built into the base is subjective, based on fitness level, speed, and total distance being swum. The following list shows the amount of rest to shoot for at various distances. Five seconds is usually the minimum that's realistic for a fitness swimmer regardless of the total distance. This amount of time allows a few deep breaths and an additional moment to find the clock, process the information, and regroup before pushing off again.

50 yards or meters—5 seconds

100 yards or meters—7 to 8 seconds

150 yards or meters—10 seconds

200 yards or meters—15 seconds

250 yards or meters—17 to 18 seconds

300 yards or meters—20 seconds

# Gauging Effort

Applying the concept of interval training to its fullest requires knowing how hard you're working at any time in the pool. Being able to exert just the right amount of effort in every set of a workout is critical to improvement. The interval in some sets will be relatively easy, others moderate, and still others quite difficult. Each set targets a specific aspect of fitness that will develop only if the exertion level is within a set range. The ability to remain within range depends largely on being in tune with your body and recognizing the effort you're exerting at any point in the session. Being this aware of the physical level at which you're working at any given time is difficult in the early stages of a new workout regimen. The extremes—swimming with virtually no effort or at an all-out sprint—are pretty easy to identify. But learning to read the signals coming from your body at the levels in between takes a little more perception. Quantifying that effort using preestablished guidelines can become second nature with time and attentiveness.

There are two primary methods of identifying exertion level: heart rate and an effort scale. Each has its advantages and disadvantages. The two methods can be used individually or in conjunction with each other. Although using heart rate is the more popular method, my recommendation for fitness swimmers is to use the measures together to negate the inaccuracies and inconsistencies of each.

## Heart Rate

Heart rate is a good barometer for how hard you're working at any given time. The more challenging an activity, the more oxygen the muscles need to perform the activity. The body's solution is delivering more oxygen-carrying blood to the muscles at work, which means the heart must pump more frequently and vigorously. The number of times a heart beats per minute is commonly known as the heart rate, and the upper limit of the number of times a heart can beat in one minute is known as the maximum heart rate (MHR).

Determining MHR is difficult to do with pinpoint precision. There are several mathematical formulas to estimate a person's MHR, the most common of which is 220 minus age in years. None is completely accurate because of the many variables among different populations. The most accurate formula, as concluded in a 2003 study published in the *Journal of Exercise Physiology*, is 205.8 – (.685 × age) (Robergs and Landwehr 2002).

A physical test is the best way to determine an individual's MHR, but even that is subjective. Regardless of the activity, a person must already have a fitness base for that activity before an MHR test can be exact. Maximum heart rates vary according to the activity, so your MHR when running likely won't be your MHR when swimming. Also, because age and fitness level alter the MHR, performing the test every two to three months is necessary to keep the rate current. The complexity and length of the test also should vary depending on the fitness and competitiveness of the swimmer. For the purposes of this book, performing the following test on a day when you're feeling fresh and strong should provide results with sufficient accuracy. Be warned, though: The test is physically challenging if done properly.

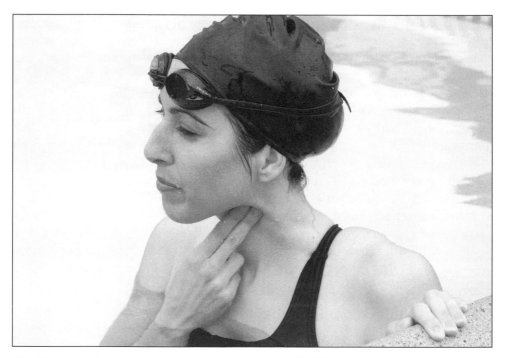

Checking your heart rate at the end of a main set is helpful in determining your exertion level.

After warming up for about 10 minutes, swim 400 yards or meters as quickly as you can, including the last 50 all-out. This test might take some practice to learn how hard to swim in the first 350 to have enough gas in your tank to really kick it up a notch in the last 50. Take your pulse for 10 seconds immediately after finishing. That number multiplied by six is your maximum heart rate. Cool down for 10 minutes (Sleamaker and Browning 1996).

Once you know how to calculate your MHR, you can apply this measurement to your workout. Using heart rate to gauge effort involves swimming at varying percentages of your MHR depending on the nature of the set or type of workout. Those percentages are called the target heart rate (THR) zones. Determining the heart rate zones in which you should swim at specific times in a workout is only a matter of math. Simply multiply your MHR by the percentage of intensity a set in a workout calls for. For example, the THR zone of a person with an MHR of 178 swimming a warm-up set (55 to 60 percent of MHR) should be between 98 and 107.

This method is a very personal gauge for exertion level because of the many factors that affect MHR. In addition to the ones already mentioned, overall fitness level, gender, and energy level during a workout also affect MHR. On average, a fit person will have a higher MHR than an unfit person; a swimmer will have a higher MHR in the pool than a nonswimmer will have; a younger person's MHR will be higher than that of an older person; and a male's MHR is higher than a female's. These are generalities, and many individuals' MHR will go against the averages. However, MHR also varies for an individual depending on a variety of factors, such as rest, nutrition, hydration, energy level, age, and fitness levels, so using only MHR to measure effort even for an individual is somewhat subjective.

## Effort Scale

Although heart rate appears to offer quantifiable evidence of how hard you're working, the variables among and within individuals make this method by no means perfect. I strongly recommend that fitness swimmers either use an effort scale (ES) alone or in conjunction with heart rate to help identify the difficulty of each swim set or workout. Because ES is based on how hard it feels you are working during any point in the workout, the scale is universally applicable on any given day. However, this method is not perfect because of its subjectivity. Identifying the feeling of how hard you are working takes practice and commitment to increase consistency and accuracy.

Table 3.1 classifies ES based on a scale of 1 to 10 and on the more common activity of walking and running. The table lists each level by difficulty, effort level, on-land example, and target heart rate based on a percentage of MHR. An ES of 1 in the swimming pool is extremely easy, equating to a slow saunter on land. An ES of 10 in the swimming pool is extremely difficult, equating to an all-out sprint on land.

## Table 3.1    Effort Scale

| ES | Difficulty | Effort level | Example | THR |
|----|-----------|--------------|---------|-----|
| 1 | Extremely easy | Very little effort | Slow saunter | 55% |
| 2 | Very easy | Little effort | Saunter | 60% |
| 3 | Somewhat easy | Some effort | Normal walk | 65% |
| 4 | Moderate | Moderate effort | Brisk walk | 70% |
| 5 | Becoming demanding | Definite effort | Jog | 75% |
| 6 | Somewhat demanding | Significant effort | Moderate jog | 80% |
| 7 | Demanding | Serious effort | Run | 85% |
| 8 | Difficult | Very serious effort | Fast run | 90% |
| 9 | Very difficult | Near-maximal effort | Near sprint | 95% |
| 10 | Extremely difficult | Maximal effort | All-out sprint | 100% |

New swimmers often have some difficulty in using ES. Those who are learning to swim or who are in the very beginning stages of swimming for fitness, regardless of fitness level on land, will find almost any pace in the pool difficult. The information earlier in this chapter on building swim fitness, as well as the workouts in chapter 5, will help new swimmers build their aerobic endurance to the point at which they can use ES or heart rate to identify workout zones. But regardless of experience or fitness level, learning to recognize and swim each effort level will bring the greatest gains in your fitness and performances.

# Injury Prevention

Swimming is about as easy on the body as any exercise activity can be. Warming up, cooling down, and stretching are by far the best ways to prevent injuries. Allowing muscles, ligaments, tendons, and joints to loosen up fully before going hard in a workout and then stretching them out in the cool-down afterward keeps the vast majority of potential injuries from developing.

Still, there are two areas of the body that can develop pain if not taken care of properly: the shoulders and the knees. The most prevalent are shoulder problems caused almost exclusively in fitness swimmers by a lack of sufficient warm-up, overuse, or not being accustomed to certain strokes. Whenever you feel any amount of pain or twinge when you are swimming, pulling, or drilling, the best course of action is to stop swimming immediately—not when you finish a length or lap or set, but right away. Float on

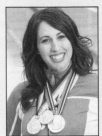

# Swimming While Pregnant

Swimming has been a part of my life for literally longer than I can remember. I was 18 months old when I first started swimming, was doing laps at 2 years old, and began competing when I was 5. I have no memory of not swimming.

So when I became pregnant with my first child, the thought of stopping swimming never entered my mind. And it shouldn't have, because swimming is one of the best ways for a pregnant woman to stay healthy—for herself and her child—during the months leading up to delivery. Swimming is low impact, so it doesn't make the body ache or overjostle the baby. Moderate swims don't elevate the heart rate to the extent that running does, so the baby isn't deprived of oxygen. And in the later stages of the pregnancy, when getting comfortable on land becomes increasingly difficult, the ability to fully stretch out in the buoyancy of the water can be quite soothing. You don't feel heavy, and you feel that your baby has plenty of room to stretch out.

The only caveat is that you have to slow down virtually from the moment you know you're pregnant, even before you start to show. The physiological changes in the body are astounding and taxing from the very beginning. Competitive or experienced swimmers no longer will be able to swim as fast as they had just weeks before. Flip turns should be abandoned, and rest within and between sets will expand to periods that might be embarrassing to mention to your swimming buddies. That's okay. Such effects should be as expected as the growing size of your belly. The pressure to perform or improve should be replaced by the joy of knowing that simply swimming laps is keeping you and your baby fit and healthy. Who knows, swimming pregnant might even give your baby a head start in the pool!

your back and kick to the end of the pool, and get out of the water so you don't aggravate a possible injury. If you stop your workout short that day, and if you have suffered an injury, you'll be back in the water much sooner than if you try to gut it out. Stretch your shoulders out really well and ice them for 15 to 20 minutes at a time two or three times a day. After one or two days of rest, gently swing your arm forward and backward. If you feel no pain at all, get back in the pool, after a thorough stretching session, and swim a couple of easy laps at ES 1 to test things out. If there's no pain, continue warming up very gradually, and spend the majority of the workout stretching out at a fairly low intensity. Jumping back into an intense set the first day back might re-strain the muscle and cause further time missed in the pool.

The other injury that occurs with some regularity is to the knees when swimming breaststroke, especially if the kick is not done properly. Follow the procedure as just described: stop swimming immediately, stretch your hamstrings and quadriceps, ice the knee, and rest a day or two. Get back in the water after the pain is gone, and warm up slowly and thoroughly before beginning an easy workout.

# chapter 4

# Stretching, Core Strengthening, and Drills

Elite swimmers' daily regimens at the pool involve more than just swimming. Two other important aspects of a complete swim workout that maximize the benefits of swimming while minimizing the chance of injury are stretching the major muscles of the body and strengthening its core. The value of flexibility and core muscle strength—both in swimming and in life—is hard to overstate. A limber body allows for a longer stretch during the swimming strokes, which improves efficiency. Elasticity also provides a sort of safeguard if the body is ever overextended by enabling the body to more fully adapt to the unusual or overloaded positions in which we sometimes put ourselves. This cuts down on both tweaks and full-blown injuries.

As you read in chapter 2, core strength is critical to proper execution of any swimming stroke. Strong hip, abdominal, and back muscles keep the body in the most efficient position throughout the stroke, thus reducing drag and increasing performance. In this chapter we'll look at exercises included in two preworkout routines that will keep your body flexible and core muscles strong.

Also covered in this chapter are 19 effective yet straightforward drills to improve the efficiency of your stroke. Swimming is good exercise, regardless of your form. But improving technique in each stroke will yield fitness and performance benefits. Drilling each stroke is by far the best way to make improvements. Each of the drills for the freestyle, backstroke, breaststroke, and butterfly are included in at least one workout in part II, with those for freestyle appearing most. Don't hesitate to spend extra time working on drills. The results make the effort well worth it.

# Preworkout Routines

Many beginning and intermediate swimmers skimp on preworkout routines. On the surface, stretching and core work can feel as if they are taking up valuable time that could be spent doing more "quality" laps in a workout. These swimmers want to get in the water, do their intervals or laps, and be done with it. But adding in the time for exercises before getting in the pool is more valuable in the long run than an extra dozen laps.

Along with the routines I'll describe in this chapter, if you choose to run, cycle, lift weights, or do any other type of exercise on the same day as your swim workout, I recommend doing those before swimming as well. Swimming elongates the body much more than any exercise other than yoga. Making swimming the last physical activity of the day helps stretch out the muscles and finish with low-impact exercise.

## Stretching

Consider stretching to be the first phase of a workout rather than an optional prelude. Stretching not only loosens up the body in preparation for the demands placed on it in the pool, it also allows the mind to begin shifting from the details of real life to the details of the workout. Perhaps the best part of stretching is how good it feels. The first week or so might be uncomfortable if you're new to stretching, but it doesn't take long before it feels as if you're bending or squeezing out the body's tensions. Even so, swimmers often have a hard time making themselves stretch before getting in the water. Along with lack of time or simply not wanting to build it into the workout, a common excuse is that there's no natural place to stretch at the pool. Throughout my career, I stretched poolside on my towel, and I've continued to do so as I swim for fitness.

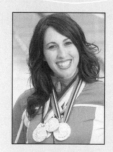

## Enjoying Stretching

Throughout my career, stretching was an integral part of my workout each day, and I truly believe it played an important role in my success. But even knowing that at the time, it wasn't the prime motivating factor in my being so consistent with the routine. Those 10 to 15 minutes on the pool deck were such an enjoyable part of my day, providing a perfect time to transition from the chaos of the day to the focus required of my time in the pool. My teammates and I used the time to catch up on each others' lives, talk about how we felt going into the workout, and in general take advantage of the last moments of serenity before starting another tough workout.

The stretching routine I'll share with you enabled me to swim at the highest level for more than 10 years without a significant injury. This routine will help you prevent muscle strains and pulls so you can swim as often as you like. A full description of each stretch follows the routine. Swimming is all about flexibility, so it's important to be loosened up before getting in the water. If you hold each stretch 10 to 15 seconds and perform each exercise 10 to 15 times, the routine takes no more than 10 minutes. At the end of the stretch routine, shake it out! Stand up straight and shake the head, arms, torso, and each leg to finish loosening up the body.

---

### Stretching Routine

Double-arm swing stretch forward

Double-arm swing stretch backward

Single-arm swing stretch forward (right arm)

Single-arm swing stretch forward (left arm)

Single-arm swing stretch backward (right arm)

Single-arm swing stretch backward (left arm)

Double-arm swing stretch cross-body

Cross-body stretch (right arm)

Cross-body stretch (left arm)

Down-spine stretch (right arm)

Down-spine stretch (left arm)

Streamline stretch

Standing toe-touch stretch (middle)

Standing toe-touch stretch (right foot)

Standing toe-touch stretch (left foot)

Sitting toe-touch stretch

Sitting hurdle stretch (right leg)

Sitting hurdle stretch (left leg)

Groin stretch

Ankle circle stretch (clockwise)

Ankle circle stretch (counterclockwise)

Neck stretch

Head circles (clockwise)

Head circles (counterclockwise)

Shake it out!

---

## Arm Swing Stretches

You can swing your arms in a variety of ways to get a good, overall stretch in your arms. You can swing both arms at the same time or one at a time, and you can change the direction of your swing. For a double-arm swing stretch forward, stand up straight, keep both arms straight, and swing them concurrently in as large a forward circle as your shoulder rotation allows without the hands crossing in front of the body. For a double-arm swing stretch backward, reverse the direction of the circle.

For a single-arm swing stretch, stand up straight and keep the active arm straight as you swing it in as large a forward circle as your shoulder rotation allows without letting the hand cross in front of the body (figure 4.1a). Keep your inactive arm relaxed by your side. Alternate active and inactive arms, and swing each arm both forward and backward.

The final variation is a double-arm swing stretch across the body. Stand up straight, keep both arms straight, and swing them concurrently in as large a diagonal forward circle as your shoulder rotation allows. Hands should cross in front of the body (figure 4.1b).

## Cross-Body Stretch

To stretch the right arm, stand up straight and use the left forearm to pull the right elbow toward the body. The right arm should remain horizontal to the ground, and the right elbow should wind up near the left shoulder (figure 4.2). The stretch should be felt in the muscles just below the right shoulder. To stretch the left arm, do the opposite.

## Down-Spine Stretch

To stretch the right arm, stand up straight, point the right elbow to the sky, and place the right hand in the middle of the upper back. Use the left hand to push the elbow back so the right hand moves down the spine (figure 4.3). The stretch should be felt in the right triceps and the muscles just below the right shoulder. To stretch the left arm, do the opposite.

## Streamline Stretch

Standing up straight with arms straight, put hands above the head in a streamline position. Stand tiptoe and elongate the entire body as far as you can (figure 4.4). The stretch should be felt through the legs, torso, shoulders, and arms.

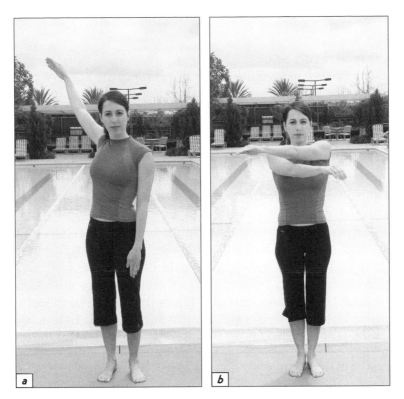

**Figure 4.1** *(a)* Single-arm swing stretch; *(b)* double-arm swing stretch cross-body.

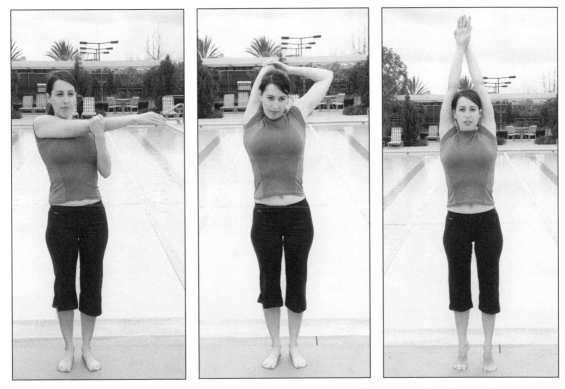

**Figure 4.2** Cross-body stretch.     **Figure 4.3** Down-spine stretch.     **Figure 4.4** Streamline stretch.

## Toe-Touch Stretch

Toe-touch stretches can be done either standing or sitting. For the standing toe-touch stretch, stand up straight with feet shoulder-width apart, bend at the waist, and touch the toes on both feet with the fingers or palms of both hands. Keep hands side by side and legs straight. The stretch should be felt in the hips and down the backs of both legs.

You also can stretch the muscles that run up the sides of the hips and legs by bending to touch the toes on either the right or left foot. Stand up straight with feet shoulder-width apart. To stretch the left side, bend at the waist and touch the left toes with the fingers or palms of both hands. Keep hands side by side and legs straight (figure 4.5a). The stretch should be felt in the hips and down the backs of both legs, with slightly more emphasis on the left side. To stretch the right side, do the opposite.

For a sitting toe-touch stretch, sit on a level surface with legs straight in front of you. Lean at the waist and touch the toes of both feet with both hands (figure 4.5b). If possible, continue leaning and try to touch your nose to your knees. The stretch should be felt in the hips and down the backs of both legs.

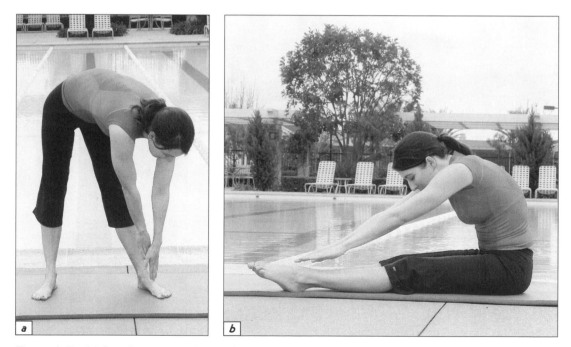

**Figure 4.5** (a) Standing toe-touch stretch to one side, and (b) sitting toe-touch stretch.

## Sitting Hurdle Stretch

To stretch the right leg, sit on a level surface with the right leg straight in front of you. Bend the left leg and place the left foot on the inside of the right thigh. Lean at the waist and try to touch the nose to the right knee (figure 4.6). The stretch should be felt in the hips, down the back of the right leg, and on the left side of the back. To stretch the left leg, do the opposite.

## Groin Stretch

Sitting on a level surface, bend both legs so that the bottoms of both feet are touching right in front of the body. Press knees down toward the ground with hands or elbows (figure 4.7). The stretch should be felt along the inside thighs of both legs.

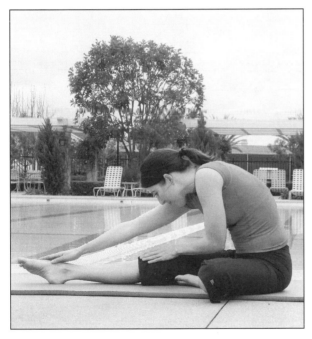

**Figure 4.6**  Sitting hurdle stretch.

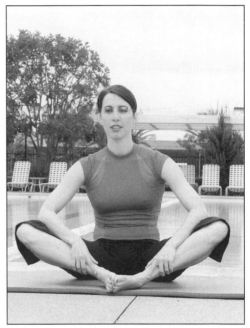

**Figure 4.7**  Groin stretch.

## Ankle Circle Stretch

Sitting on a level surface with both legs bent at 90-degree angles, cross one leg over the other and draw imaginary circles in the air with the toes (figure 4.8). The stretch should be felt in the lower legs and ankles and performed both clockwise and counterclockwise.

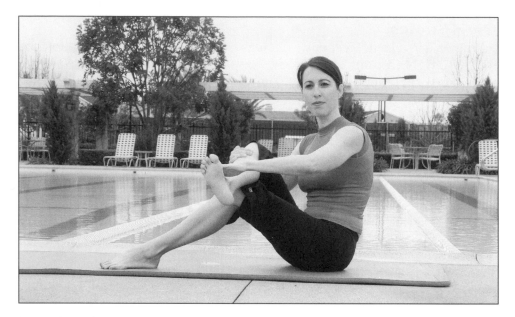

**Figure 4.8**   Ankle circle stretch.

## Neck Stretch

Sitting up straight, bend the neck forward so the chin touches the chest, then back so the chin points toward the sky, then to the left so the left ear is near the left shoulder, and finally to the right so the right ear is near the right shoulder. Then move the head in slow, controlled circles, both clockwise and counterclockwise. The stretch should be felt in the neck on the opposite side of the direction in which the head is leaning (figure 4.9).

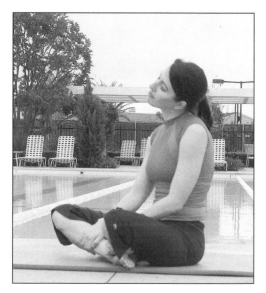

**Figure 4.9**   Neck stretch.

# Core Strengthening

Core strengthening is another phase of the workout that tends to be skipped, but it can help you tremendously with your technique in the water. The following routine is similar to the one my teammates and I did before every workout. If possible, this routine should be done right after stretching and before getting in the water. Otherwise, in the morning right after waking up or at night just before bed are also good times to get core work in.

The first five exercises are done individually, followed by two optional exercises if you have a training partner. Begin by doing 15 repetitions of each exercise with little to no rest between each, and try to build up until you're doing 25 reps each. You might be amazed at what a difference you'll feel in the pool. The routine should take about five minutes. If you believe that a lack of core strength is hindering your swimming progress, consider supplementing your swimming workouts with yoga or Pilates. Both forms of exercise are phenomenal for building core strength, and yoga includes the added benefit of greatly improving flexibility.

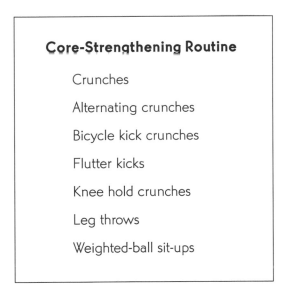

**Core-Strengthening Routine**

Crunches

Alternating crunches

Bicycle kick crunches

Flutter kicks

Knee hold crunches

Leg throws

Weighted-ball sit-ups

## Crunches

Lying flat on the back on a flat, soft surface, lift and bend the legs with thighs perpendicular to the ground, knees above hips, and lower legs parallel to the ground. Touch the sides of the head with the fingertips so that the elbows point toward the knees. Flex the abdominal muscles to raise the upper torso in a smooth manner until both shoulder blades are off the ground (figure 4.10). Immediately return to the ground and repeat. Be careful not to allow the fingers to drift back and pull the neck forward. The neck muscles should engage to keep the head in a neutral position throughout the crunch.

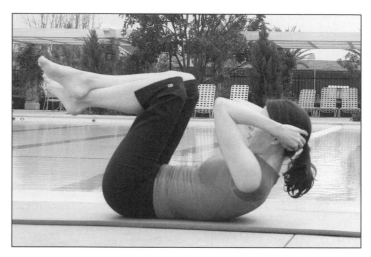

**Figure 4.10**   Crunches.

## Alternating Crunches

Lying flat on the back on a flat, soft surface, lift and bend both legs with thighs perpendicular to the ground, knees above hips, and lower legs parallel to the ground. Touch the sides of the head with the fingertips so that elbows point toward the knees. Flex the abdominal muscles to raise the upper torso in a smooth manner until shoulder blades are off the ground. At the same time, contract the internal and external oblique muscles to touch the right elbow to the left knee (figure 4.11). Immediately return to the ground and repeat, this time touching the left elbow to the right knee. Count each elbow-to-knee touch as one repetition. Be careful not to allow the fingers to drift back and pull the neck forward. The neck muscles should engage to keep the head in a neutral position throughout the crunch.

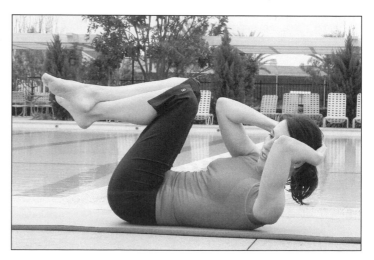

**Figure 4.10**   Alternating crunches.

## Bicycle Kick Crunches

Bicycle kick crunches are like alternating crunches except the legs are moving in a pedaling motion at the same time. Lie flat on the back on a flat, soft surface. Lift both legs so they hover about six inches (15 centimeters) off the ground. Touch the sides of the head with the fingertips so that elbows point toward knees. Flex the abdominal muscles to raise the upper torso in a smooth manner until shoulder blades are off the ground, as if doing an alternating crunch. At the same time, contract the internal and external oblique muscles to bring the right elbow into the position it would be in to touch the left knee if doing alternating crunches (figure 4.12). While raising the torso, bring the left knee up to meet the right elbow. The right leg should be moving to a straight position. Immediately lower the torso to the ground and straighten the left leg; do the same with the opposite elbow and leg. At no time should either leg stop moving or touch the ground. Count each elbow-to-knee touch as one repetition. Take care that the fingers don't drift back and pull the neck forward. The neck muscles should engage to keep the head in a neutral position throughout the exercise.

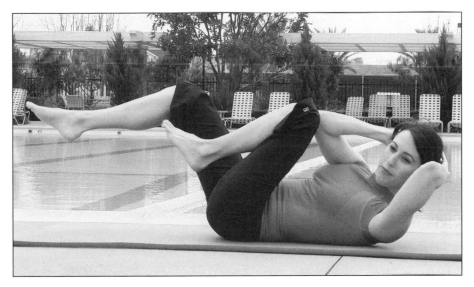

**Figure 4.12** Bicycle kick crunches.

## Flutter Kicks

Lying flat on the back on a flat, soft surface, place hands underneath the bottom with palms on the ground and stretch the legs out long and straight in a streamline position. Lift both legs off the ground about six inches (15 centimeters) and begin to flutter kick as quickly as possible (figure 4.13). While alternately moving the legs up and down, initiate the kick with the hips, relax the ankles, and keep the knees bent slightly. Count one repetition when both legs have kicked once.

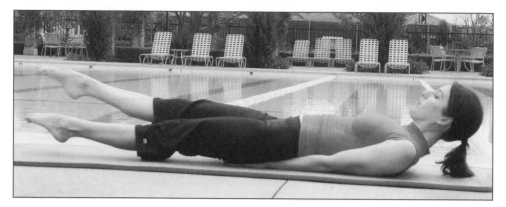

**Figure 4.13**   Flutter kick exercise.

## Knee Hold Crunches

Lie flat on the back on a flat, soft surface, with hands underneath the bottom and the legs stretched out long and straight in a streamline position. Start with the legs hovering about six inches (15 centimeters) about the ground (figure 4.14a), and then pull the knees tight to the chest by using your abdominal muscles (4.14b). Hold for five seconds, then slowly return legs to the streamline position about six inches (15 centimeters) above the ground. Count each pull as one repetition.

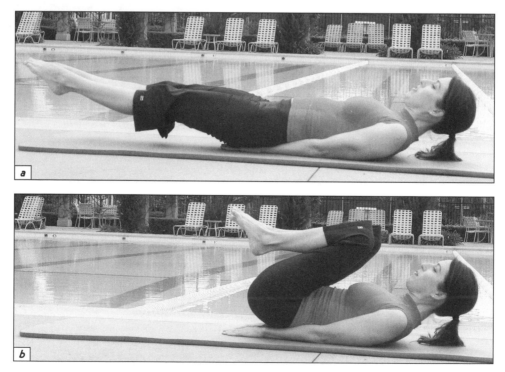

**Figure 4.14**   Knee hold crunch: *(a)* legs straight and *(b)* legs bent to chest.

## Leg Throws

This exercise requires two people. The exerciser lies faceup on a flat, soft surface, holding on to her partner's ankles, with her legs as straight and long as possible about six inches (15 centimeters) off the ground in a modified streamline position. The partner stands at the exerciser's head. The exerciser performs a straight-leg lift using the hip and abdominal muscles until legs are straight above the head and perpendicular to the ground (figure 4.15a). The partner pushes the exerciser's legs back toward the ground with enough force that the exerciser must reengage the hip and abdominal muscles to return the legs to the modified streamline position without them hitting the ground (figure 4.15b). The difficulty for the exerciser is in "catching" the legs before they hit the ground. The exerciser's legs should be in continuous motion; the partner should alternate pushing the legs to each side and the middle.

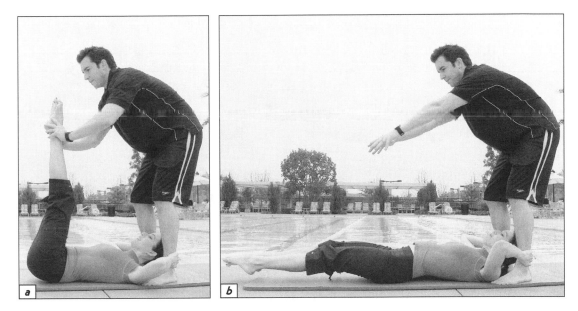

**Figure 4.15** Leg throws.

## Weighted-Ball Sit-Ups

This exercise requires two people and a weighted exercise ball. Both people lie on the ground with their knees interlocked at about a 45-degree angle. The person with the medicine ball sits up and throws the ball to the partner while finishing the upward motion (figure 4.16a). The partner catches the ball while beginning a downward motion (figure 4.16b). The partners should move in a seesaw motion, developing a rhythm with the ball exchange. Count one repetition when both partners have done one sit-up.

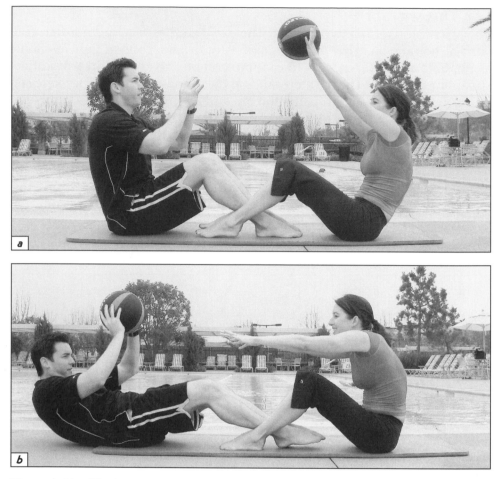

**Figure 4.16** Weighted-ball sit-ups: (a) throwing the ball and (b) partner catching the ball.

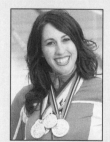

# 1,000 Sit-Ups,
# Usually Twice a Day

When I was swimming competitively, each season we would work up to doing 10 to 15 continuous minutes of core strengthening exercises before every workout. There were 10 different exercises in our routine, including the ones just described, and we would build up to doing 100 repetitions of each exercise in rapid succession. Your math is correct—that adds up to 1,000 abdominal exercises! But usually that was only half of it. For most of my career I swam twice a day, and we'd go through the routine before both workouts. There's a reason elite swimmers' bellies are flat!

# Workout Drills

Dozens and dozens of drills have been developed to refine the four main swimming strokes. The 20 drills included here are useful for any swimmer who wants to improve technique. Although the drills are easy enough for less experienced swimmers to execute properly, they also provide excellent stroke-refinement opportunities for even the most elite swimmers. When these drills are included in a workout, they are often followed by a normal lap of swimming. That lap is not intended as a break from thinking about the stroke. On the contrary, you should focus on the feel of the previous drill during the lap to fine-tune your stroke. Four of the drills—Sidekick, 10-10 Kick, One-Arm, 3-3-3, and Fist—are used for more than one stroke, with technique tailored to the particular stroke. Sidekick, 10-10 Kick, and Fist are the least complicated of the drills in the book. One-Arm is a straightforward drill—swimming with one arm at a time—and 3-3-3 is a variation thereof.

## Freestyle Stroke Drills

These six drills are among my very favorites—both to share with others and to swim in practice myself—because they are so effective at focusing on different aspects of the freestyle stroke. Freestyle Sidekick Drill and Freestyle 10-10 Kick Drill emphasize the rotation of the body. Freestyle One Arm Drill is essentially swimming the freestyle normally but with only one arm stroking. Freestyle 3-3-3 Drill is a variation of Freestyle One-Arm Drill. Freestyle Fist Drill stresses the backward-S path the hands and forearms follow when underwater, and Freestyle Hip-Shoulder-Forehead Drill puts the arm at an angle that forces the body to rotate and the hand to enter the water at the optimal angle to begin the next stroke.

### FREESTYLE SIDEKICK DRILL

**Goal:** To simulate the angled position the body should be in as it rotates from one side to the other

**Execution:** From the streamline position, stretch the left arm out as far as possible and turn the body to between a 45- and 60-degree angle to the surface of the water. The left earlobe should be against the left shoulder so that you're looking toward the right side of the pool. Place the right arm down against the right side of the body, where it remains throughout the drill, and flutter kick (figure 4.17). Whenever you need to breathe, simply turn the head upward a few inches (or a dozen centimeters), which lifts the mouth out of the water. Take a little breath, and return the head to the same position.

**Gold Medal Advice:** This drill is great for helping the body experience how it feels to kick in an angled position, which is beneficial because in freestyle the body is parallel to the bottom of the pool for only a very short time. Be sure to perform the drill equally on both sides to keep the body balanced in its feel for the water.

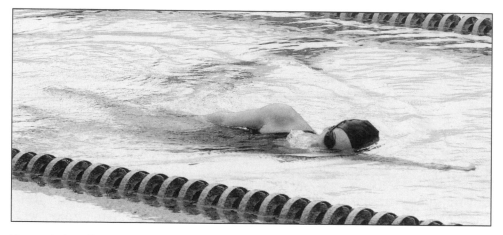

**Figure 4.17**   Freestyle Sidekick Drill.

## FREESTYLE 10-10 KICK DRILL

**Goal:** To focus on a 180-degree rotation of the body and executing a perfect underwater stroke during the pull part of the drill

**Execution:** Freestyle 10-10 Kick Drill is an offshoot of Freestyle Sidekick Drill. As in that drill, start in the streamline position. Stretch the right arm out as far as possible and turn the body to between a 45- and 60-degree angle to the surface of the water. Place the left arm down against the left side of the body and flutter kick 5 times with each foot for a total of 10 kicks. Then do a perfect stroke to rotate 180 degrees to the opposite side. Stretch the left arm out as far as possible, place the right arm against the right side of the body, and flutter kick another 10 times. Continue switching sides every 10 kicks throughout the drill.

**Gold Medal Advice:** You'll probably take only five or six swimming strokes during this drill.

## FREESTYLE ONE-ARM DRILL

**Goal:** To focus on arm movement during a stroke by eliminating the motion of one arm

**Execution:** To swim with the right arm, begin in streamline position and stroke with the right arm, keeping the left arm in streamline position in front of your body at all times. Make sure the right hand enters the water with a knifelike motion but does not cross the invisible line bisecting the body. With each stroke, the right arm should stretch out about a hand-length beyond the left hand to accentuate the extended position. Feet should kick normally for freestyle. To swim with the left arm, keep the right arm in the streamline position and stroke with the left arm.

**Gold Medal Advice:** Focus on the backward-S path of the stroking arm: the sweep out and sweep in to the hips and the push at the end of the stroke. Also focus on keeping the head in streamline position, with the water hitting the forehead between the eyebrows and hairline. Swim equally with each arm to stay balanced.

## FREESTYLE 3-3-3 DRILL

**Goal:** To focus on arm movement during a stroke by eliminating the motion of one arm yet getting a step closer than Freestyle One-Arm Drill to putting it all together in a normal stroke

**Execution:** Start by swimming with the right arm for three strokes, keeping the left arm in front as in Freestyle One-Arm Drill. Then swim with the left arm for three strokes. Finally, swim three full cycles, three strokes with each arm. Concentrate on the arm motion and head position throughout the drill, and continue swimming in the 3-3-3 pattern for the entire distance.

**Gold Medal Advice:** Always keep the nonstroking arm in streamline position in front of the body rather than allowing it to sink and drag.

## FREESTYLE FIST DRILL

**Goal:** To develop a feel for the water with the forearms and reinforce the path the hands take during each stroke

**Execution:** Swim freestyle normally except with the hands clinched into fists instead of straight like knife blades.

**Gold Medal Advice:** Most swimmers place almost all of their attention on their hands when swimming freestyle, not realizing the forearms are part of the stroke as well. Focus on feeling the forearm make a backward-S motion in the water.

## FREESTYLE HIP-SHOULDER-FOREHEAD DRILL

**Goal:** To reinforce proper hand position at reentry and to draw the body's attention to how it feels to swim at an angle

**Execution:** Swim the freestyle normally except for the recovery phase of each stroke. Start the recovery as usual, but when the elbow begins to leave the water, touch the fingertips to that side's hip (figure 4.18a), then shoulder (4.18b), then forehead (4.18c). The position of the hand when touching the forehead should look like a downward military salute, with fingertips pointing toward the bridge of the nose.

**Gold Medal Advice:** This is my favorite drill. Although it is the most complicated of the drills to learn, the benefits are well worth it. The arm angle from the quasi-salute forces the hand to enter the water in a near-perfect position, cut knifelike through the surface of the water, and get a clean catch. This drill also helps the arm stretch out as long as possible and allows the swimmer to feel the rotation motion of the freestyle, both of which are so important when swimming freestyle.

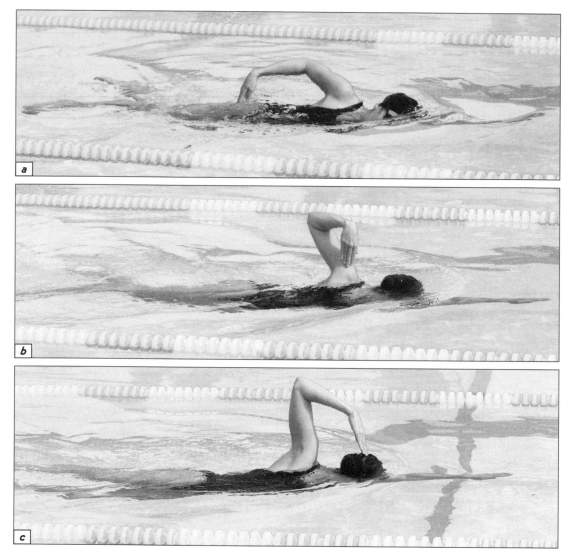

**Figure 4.18**   Freestyle Hip-Shoulder-Forehead Drill.

# Backstroke Drills

Four of the five backstroke drills are variations of the freestyle drills, but that shouldn't be surprising considering how similar the strokes are. Backstroke Sidekick Drill and Backstroke 10-10 Kick Drill emphasize the rotation of the body, particularly getting the shoulder to the chin and keeping the core flexed and hips up. The isolation created in Backstroke One-Arm Drill and Backstroke 3-3-3 Drill makes you concentrate on upper-body mechanics and the pinkie leading the hand into the water. Backstroke Steady Head Drill is a fun balancing drill that promotes keeping the head straight throughout the stroke.

## BACKSTROKE SIDEKICK DRILL

**Goal:** To simulate the angled position the body should be in as it rotates from one side to the other

**Execution:** From the inverted streamline position in which the backstroke is swum, stretch the right arm out as far as possible so that the right hand is in the entry position (pinkie finger first). Take care not to cross the invisible line that bisects the body. Put the left hand down on the left hip and turn the body to between a 45- and 60-degree angle to the water's surface. The right shoulder should be angled down in the water and the left shoulder angled up out of the water, touching the chin. Flutter kick from that stretched out, angled position (figure 4.19).

**Gold Medal Advice:** Make sure the right shoulder is almost directly behind the head, the left shoulder is literally touching the chin, and the head is perfectly straight in an inverted streamline position. Perform the drill equally on both sides to keep the body balanced in its feel for the water.

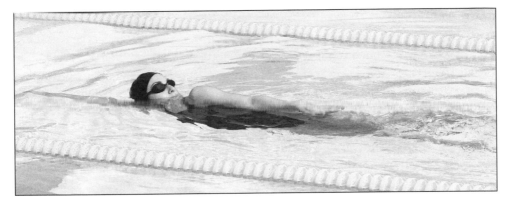

**Figure 4.19**   Backstroke Sidekick Drill.

## BACKSTROKE 10-10 KICK DRILL

**Goal:** To focus on the 180-degree rotation of the body and to execute a perfect underwater stroke during the pull part of the drill

**Execution:** This drill is an offshoot of Backstroke Sidekick Drill. Just as in that drill, start in the streamline position. Stretch the right arm out as far as possible and turn the body to between a 45- and 60-degree angle to the surface of the water. Place the left arm down against the left side of the body and flutter kick 5 times with each foot for a total of 10 kicks. Then do a perfect stroke to rotate 180 degrees to the opposite side. Stretch the left arm out as far as possible, place the right arm against the right side of the body, and flutter kick another 10 times. Continue switching sides every 10 kicks throughout the drill.

**Gold Medal Advice:** You will probably take only about five or six swimming strokes during this drill.

## BACKSTROKE ONE-ARM DRILL

**Goal:** To focus on the upper-body movement during a stroke by eliminating the motion of one arm

**Execution:** To swim with the right arm, place the left hand down by the left hip and stroke with the right arm. Accentuate the stretch of the shoulder once the hand has entered the water. The right shoulder meets the chin with each stroke as the right arm begins to lift out of the water, and the left shoulder pops out of the water to meet the chin just as the right arm is beginning its elbow bend underneath the water. To swim with the left arm, keep the right hand next to the right hip and stroke with the left arm.

**Gold Medal Advice:** Make sure the pinky side leads the hand into the water in a choplike motion and does not cross the invisible line. Concentrate on the bend in the elbow, the pull phase of the stroke, the elbow angle when it touches the ribs, and the push of the hand past the hips. Swim equally with each arm to stay balanced.

## BACKSTROKE 3-3-3 DRILL

**Goal:** To focus on upper-body movement during a stroke by eliminating the motion of one arm, yet getting a step closer than Backstroke One-Arm Drill to putting it all together in a normal stroke

**Execution:** Swim with your right arm for three strokes, keeping the left arm at your side. Then swim with the left arm for three strokes, keeping the right arm at your side. Finally, swim three full cycles, three strokes with each arm. Concentrate on the arm motion, the motion of getting the chin to the shoulder, and the head position throughout the drill.

**Gold Medal Advice:** Keep the nonstroking arm close along the side of the body rather than allowing it to sink and drag.

## BACKSTROKE STEADY HEAD DRILL

**Goal:** To emphasize keeping the head in proper position while swimming backstroke

**Execution:** Balance a pair of goggles (straps and all), a coin, or a small paper cup full of water on your forehead when in the inverted streamline position. Swim the backstroke normally. If the backstroke is swum with perfect head position, the object remains on the forehead (figure 4.20).

**Gold Medal Advice:** Keep the head in an inverted streamline position. Swimmers sometimes try to keep the object on their foreheads by holding the head up and straining their necks. This makes the drill easier but doesn't help your backstroke technique.

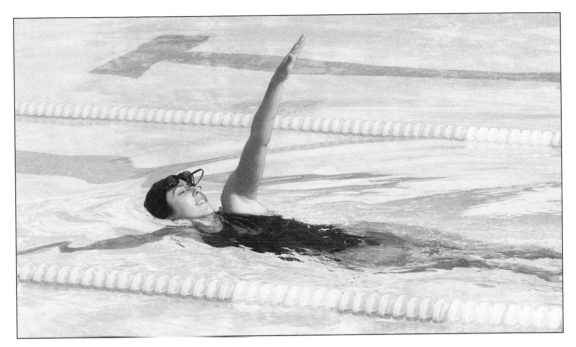

**Figure 4.20** Backstroke Steady Head Drill.

# Breaststroke Drills

Of the five breaststroke drills, two target the kick, two target upper-body movement, and one puts it all together by focusing on the timing. Both Breaststroke Heels-to-Fingertips Drill and Breaststroke Up-Out-Together Drill reinforce the Up phase of the kick with flexed ankles, the only difference being the position of the arms. Breaststroke One-Arm Drill and Breaststroke Fist Drill do the same for this stroke as the others, respectively, narrowing the focus of the arm action and providing a new way to feel the hand and arm path. Finally, Breaststroke 3-2-1 Drill develops the timing necessary to start and finish the movements of the upper and lower body simultaneously.

## BREASTSTROKE HEELS-TO-FINGERTIPS DRILL

**Goal:** To emphasize the Up motion of the breaststroke kick

**Execution:** Place each hand on its corresponding side of your bottom, with the backs of the hands touching your bottom and palms facing up toward the surface of the water. Execute the kick for the breaststroke, touching heels to fingertips in the Up phase before moving to the Out and Together phases (figure 4.21).

**Gold Medal Advice:** Remember to move the legs symmetrically and keep the ankles at 90-degree angles throughout the kick to maximize power transfer from the legs to the water.

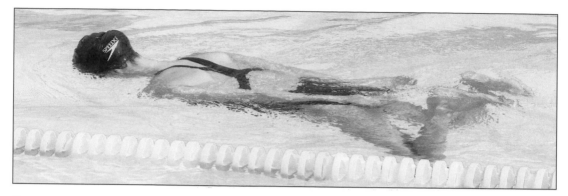

**Figure 4.21** Breaststroke Heels-to-Fingertips Drill.

## BREASTSTROKE UP-OUT-TOGETHER DRILL

**Goal:** To focus on each phase of the kick, keeping ankles flexed, and moving legs symmetrically

**Execution:** The only difference between this drill and the Breaststroke Heels-to-Fingertips Drill is the position of the arms, which are in streamline position rather than behind the back. Execute the kick for the breaststroke, touching the heels to the bottom in the Up phase before moving to the Out and Together phases (figure 4.22). Gently raise your head above water when you need to take a breath.

**Gold Medal Advice:** Breaststroke Up-Out-Together Drill builds on Breaststroke Heels-to-Fingertips Drill and should be practiced immediately afterward. After feeling the Up phase end at the fingertips in Breaststroke Heels-to-Fingertips Drill, focus on that same motion but with the upper body a bit closer to its normal position for the stroke.

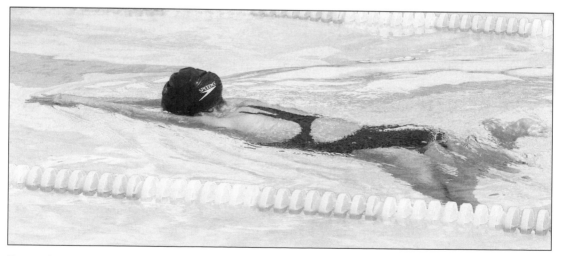

**Figure 4.22** Breaststroke Up-Out-Together Drill.

## BREASTSTROKE 3-2-1 DRILL

**Goal:** To improve the timing of the breaststroke kick and upper-body movement

**Execution:** From streamline position, kick three times and then perform one normal breaststroke stroke incorporating both the upper body and the kick. Then immediately kick two times and perform a full stroke. Finally, kick one time followed by a full stroke. Repeat the 3-2-1 pattern throughout the length of the drill.

**Gold Medal Advice:** Concentrate on the feel of the upper-body motion and the kick starting and then stopping at the same time.

## BREASTSTROKE ONE-ARM DRILL

**Goal:** To focus on arm movement during a stroke by eliminating the motion of one arm

**Execution:** To swim with the right arm, put the left arm in streamline position and stroke with the right arm. Move the fingertips along the inside lip of the imaginary bowl. Squeeze the elbow into the body and keep the forearm close to the rib cage near the bottom of the circle; then shrug the shoulder to help lift the body out of the water and move the palm of the hand past the face before relaxing to let the body drop back into a modified streamline position

**Gold Medal Advice:** Although the nonstroking arm moves somewhat because of the motion of the entire upper body when swimming breaststroke, this arm is not involved in the stroke. As with the other single-arm drills, swim equally with each arm to stay balanced.

## BREASTSTROKE FIST DRILL

**Goal:** To develop a feel for the water with the forearms and reinforce the path the hands take during each stroke

**Execution:** Swim the breaststroke normally except with hands clinched into fists.

**Gold Medal Advice:** This drill will seem difficult at first, but if you swim a lap of normal breaststroke immediately following the drill, you'll notice how much it helps you understand and feel the proper breaststroke pull.

# Butterfly Drills

Four butterfly drills are included here to help with the kick, timing, and arm motion of the stroke. Butterfly Inverted Kick Drill and Butterfly Kick Drill are exactly the same except for the position of the body, with the former performed on the back instead of the belly. Butterfly One-Arm Drill and Butterfly 3-3-3 Drill help fine-tune the arm path beneath the water and the timing of the upper body with the kick.

## BUTTERFLY INVERTED KICK DRILL

**Goal:** To help swimmers notice and correct any excess knee bend

**Execution:** Perform the butterfly kick normally but in an inverted streamline position (figure 4.23). Initiate the kick with the hips, keeping the ankles relaxed and feet together the entire time. Flex the abdominal muscles to pull the hips up slightly, using the torso and lower body to continue the undulation of the torso, hips, and legs rising and sinking in the water. The knees should never break the surface of the water.

**Gold Medal Advice:** This drill capitalizes on the fact that the best way to learn the dolphin kick is on the back in supine position. This makes it is easier to see if the knees break the surface of the water. Focus on keeping the ankles relaxed and together; generate power from the lower abdominal muscles and the hips.

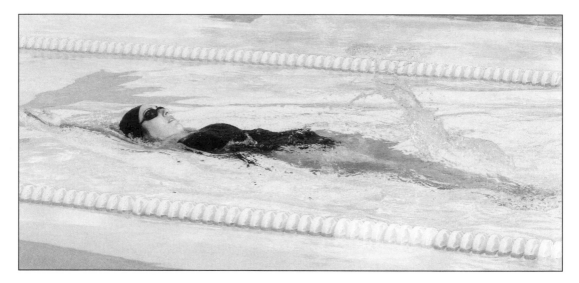

**Figure 4.23**   Butterfly Inverted Kick Drill.

## BUTTERFLY KICK DRILL

**Goal:** To develop a rhythmic and strong butterfly kick

**Execution:** Execute the butterfly kick normally but with hands at your sides (figure 4.24). Begin the kick with the hips, keeping the ankles relaxed and feet together the entire time. Use the torso and lower body to mimic the motion of a dolphin swimming through water. Flex the abdominal muscles to pull the hips up slightly, using the torso and lower body to continue the undulation of the torso, hips, and legs rising and sinking in the water.

**Gold Medal Advice:** Focus on the undulating motion of the body, keeping the ankles relaxed and together and generating power from the lower abdominal muscles and the hips.

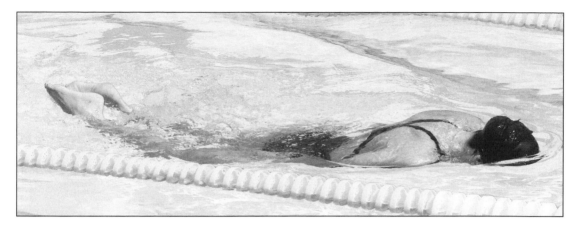

**Figure 4.24** Butterfly Kick Drill.

## BUTTERFLY ONE-ARM DRILL

**Goal:** To focus on arm movement during the butterfly stroke by eliminating the motion of one arm

**Execution:** To swim with the right arm, keep the left arm stationary in the streamline position and stroke with the right arm. The right hand should enter the water straight in front of the shoulder, thumb first. The palm then moves away from the body, back toward the belly button, and toward and past the hips, leaving the water as far down the legs as the extended arms and hands allow. To swim with the left arm, keep the right arm stationary and stroke with the left arm.

**Gold Medal Advice:** Focus on the thumb leading the hand into the water in front of the shoulder. Remember that for every butterfly stroke, there are two dolphin kicks. Swimming with a single arm helps one focus on kicking the arm back and then kicking the arm forward. Perform the drill an equal amount on each side to stay balanced.

## BUTTERFLY 3-3-3 DRILL

**Goal:** To focus on arm movement during a stroke by eliminating the motion of one arm, yet get a step closer than Butterfly One-Arm Drill to putting it all together in a normal stroke

**Execution:** Swim with the right arm for three strokes, keeping the left arm in streamline position. Then swim with your left arm for three strokes, keeping the right arm in streamline position. Finally, swim three full cycles, three strokes with each arm. Focus on the timing of the stroke with the dolphin kicks throughout the drill, and continue swimming in the 3-3-3 pattern for the entire distance.

**Gold Medal Advice:** Concentrate on synchronizing the timing of the upper body and lower body. When stroking with one arm, the nonstroking arm is in front in streamline position.

# part II

# The Workouts

In part I you have learned or had a refresher on the essentials: what equipment to tote to the pool, proper technique and drills to improve your strokes, training guidelines for swimming, and preworkout routines that can enhance life in and out of the pool. Although all that information is necessary and can pique interest in getting in the water, the real enjoyment of swimming is swimming! Gliding through the water, sensing it against your skin; using your muscles to propel you to the other end of the pool; feeling your strength, endurance, and flexibility improve each week without the wear and tear other sports can have on your body; the firmness you feel in your body after a workout; and the swimmer's high that comes once you get on a roll and workouts feel challenging yet achievable—these are the reasons swimmers swim.

The vast majority of swimmers swim in a pool as opposed to open water. Moving up and down a 25-yard or 50-meter lane at the same pace for the same number of yards or meters lap after lap, day after day, year after year might seem like the standard way to get fit in the water, matching the image of joggers running the same route at the same pace every day. But the 60 workouts in part II dispel that myth. The diversity of the workouts within and among the five categories illustrates the countless ways a pool session can be constructed to provide boredom-busting workouts that yield fitness and training benefits. You can do literally a different workout every day for the rest of your life, each one of which will help improve your health, performance, and confidence.

Twelve workouts appear in each of the five chapters—Building Swim Fitness, Building a Base, Increasing

Anaerobic Threshold, Increasing Speed, and Swimming the IM—that focus on different aspects of swim training as explained in the chapter introductions. Chapters 6, 7, and 9 begin with two workouts at 2,500 yards and progress by 500 yards for each pair, with workouts 11 and 12 at 5,000 yards. Chapter 5 begins with three workouts at 600 yards and progresses in triplets, with the final three at 2,000 yards. Chapter 8 progresses in triplets but by 500 yards, from 1,500 yards to 3,000 yards.

The workouts are constructed based on the seven sets discussed in Anatomy of a Workout (pages 59-63)—warm-up, drill set, kick set, pull set, main set, speed set, and cool-down—but not all sets are included in every workout. Although the order as just listed is the most common in which they will appear, it is altered in some workouts not only for variety but for reasons explained in the section called "Inside the Workout." This section provides a few more details about the workout, such as how to attack the various sets, what to expect as you swim them, what to focus on, and how the workout will help in your improvement as a swimmer.

Most of the workouts call for the use of at least one piece of equipment that was described as workout-enhancing gear in chapter 1. A kickboard is the most-noted gear, followed by the use of pull buoys and paddles together, then fins. Almost every pool has a rack or bin of kickboards that swimmers may use on a first-come basis. Many also have pull buoys and fins, but community paddles are relatively rare. Even if you have no equipment other than that in the mandatory category, though, you can still make excellent progress with these workouts by making the following adjustments. If you do not have access to a kickboard, kick in the streamline position, turning your head for a breath as needed; don't use fins even if the set calls for them; and slow down the interval accordingly. If you do not have a pull buoy and paddles, swim the pull sets normally, giving the workout a double-main-set feel. If you do have paddles and fins but no pull buoy, use them in the pull set but make the interval faster to reflect the aid of the fins.

Almost all intervals in the main sets of freestyle workouts are on a 1:00 per 50-yard base. This interval is very reasonable but should be altered if necessary to stay within 70 to 85 percent of your MHR. Kicking, pulling, and drill sets are a bit slower to give swimmers a chance to develop familiarity with the equipment and drills. It's important in these workouts to keep the heart rate steady and not attempt to swim too fast too soon, but at the same time you need to challenge yourself to reap the most rewards from your time in the water. Take about three minutes of rest between each set of each workout unless otherwise indicated.

If you are swimming in a 25- or 50-meter pool, as opposed to the more common 25-yard pool that these workouts are based on, you should alter the interval base in these workouts to account for the difference in length between yards and meters. Fifty yards equals 45.72 meters, or 91.4 percent of 50 yards. A good rule of thumb is to add five seconds per 50 meters when converting from yards to meters. Instead of a base of 1:00 per 50 yards, you would use a base of 1:05 per 50 meters. If you are swimming in a 50-meter pool, stop at the halfway mark when the workout calls for swimming 25 yards. Similarly, when swimming the 100 IM workouts in chapter 9, switch strokes at the halfway mark.

Swim workouts have their own language and notations that are important to understand on paper and verbally to be most comfortable following them on your own or as part of a team. Below is a compilation of sets from several different workouts in the book. After each is an explanation of how to execute the set in the pool and how to "read" the set verbally.

**Example 1**

Warm-Up (ES 1)          500 yards

1 × 100 freestyle with 20 seconds rest
1 × 75 freestyle with 15 seconds rest
1 × 50 freestyle with 10 seconds rest
1 × 25 freestyle with 5 seconds rest
*Repeat 2 times*

This 500-yard warm-up should be swum at an ES 1, classified as extremely easy. The first line means that you will swim 100 yards one time and then rest for 20 seconds at the wall. Immediately after that 20 seconds you'll swim 75 yards one time and then rest for 15 seconds. After the swims of 50 yards and 25 yards and their respective rests, "Repeat 2 times" means you will swim the set one more time.

**Example 2**

Kick Set (ES 4-5)          600 yards

Using a board and fins
8 × 75 on 2:30
Odd 75s—freestyle
Even 75s—butterfly

Any equipment to be used in the kick set will be indicated on the first line. If no equipment is to be used, the first line will start with the instruction for total distance. This set calls for swimming 75 yards eight times, leaving the wall every 2:30. The odd-numbered times you leave the wall, you will swim freestyle. The even-numbered times you leave the wall, you will swim butterfly.

**Example 3**

Pull Set (ES 5-6)          800 yards

8 × 100
#s 1-4—freestyle on 2:10
#s 5-8—freestyle on 2:05

All pull sets will use paddles and a pull buoy unless otherwise indicated. For this set, the first four of the eight 100s will be swum freestyle, pushing off from the wall every 2:10. The second group of four 100s will be swum freestyle, pushing off from the wall every 2:05.

**Example 4**

Drill Set (ES 3)                                                    250 yards
250 swim
First 50—Freestyle Hip-Shoulder-Forehead Drill
Second 50—freestyle swim, focusing on technique from previous drill
Third 50—Freestyle One-Arm Drill (25 right, 25 left)
Fourth 50—freestyle swim, focusing on technique from previous drill
Fifth 50—Freestyle 3-3-3 Drill
This drill set calls for a continuous swim of 250 yards with no stopping in
between, but the distance is swum in a variety of ways. During the first
50 yards, you will swim the Freestyle Hip-Shoulder-Forehead Drill. The
second 50 will be swum freestyle, with your attention on the rotation and
hand-entry angle emphasized in the preceding drill. During the third 50,
you'll swim the Freestyle One-Arm Drill, with your right arm going down
and the left arm coming back. The fourth 50 will be swimming freestyle,
again focusing on the technique emphasized in the previous drill. For the
final 50, you will swim the Freestyle 3-3-3 Drill.

**Example 5**

Main Set (ES 7)                                                    1,500 yards
15 × 100
#1—freestyle on 1:55 (ES 6)
#2—freestyle on 1:50 (ES 7)
#3—freestyle on 1:45 (ES 8)
*Repeat 5 times*
The 15 100s of this main set are broken into five minisets. The first repetition is to be swum on 1:55 at ES 6. The second is on 1:50 at ES 7, and the
third on 1:45 at ES 8. The time and effort for the fourth 100 starts over
again at 1:55 on ES 6, and so forth. Swim the miniset five times.

**Example 6**

Cool-Down (ES 1)                                                    200 yards
200 freestyle, mixing in some backstroke and breaststroke
This cool-down is another continuous swim. The majority of the distance
is swum freestyle, but some backstroke and breaststroke should also be
swum.

The prep work is complete. You have and know all that is necessary to
swim the workouts in part II. Now it's time to jump into the pool with the
swimming mind-set, ready for the physical and mental challenges ahead
of you. Some workouts will be more fun than others, but they'll all give
you amazing benefits and help you feel great if you stick with them!

# chapter 5

# Building Swim Fitness

This first group of workouts can be used in one of two ways. The workouts are primarily designed to help newer swimmers (or swimmers returning to the water after a long break) build their fitness in the water up to a level that enables them to successfully move on to the workouts in the other chapters in part II. Even very fit individuals who have not swum regularly or recently will likely need to start with these workouts to increase their ability to swim farther and at more varied paces. Accomplished swimmers may also use these workouts if they're pressed for time or recovering from an injury.

Freestyle is nearly the exclusive stroke in these workouts, although in a few instances you may choose to kick or drill another stroke. The workouts are grouped into four lengths: three at 600 yards, three at 1,000 yards, three at 1,500 yards, and three at 2,000 yards. The next logical step, then, would be to swim 2,500-yard workouts, which are the distances of the first two workouts in most of the other chapters in part II.

The effort level of these sets is based on an effort scale (ES) rather than a time scale. Because they use rest intervals instead of base intervals—which means that the amount of rest after each swim is fixed instead of the time between pushoffs from the wall being fixed—the workouts are a bit easier physically and mentally. These workouts are not intended to fully exhaust you or focus on endurance, speed, or other strokes, so please adjust the distances and rest times as needed to be challenging but not discouraging.

The distances of any one swim or repetition are kept short in this group of workouts. There are many more 25s in these sessions than you'll find in subsequent chapters. To continue challenging you to improve your level of fitness, I do increase the distances to 100s and some 150s as the workouts get longer, but the amount of rest also builds to help you complete the workout.

Several of the workouts are based on concepts used more consistently in later chapters, such as the ladder principle, descending, and active rest. Be sure to use the comments in the Inside the Workout section to help you understand the session.

For these workouts, the time it takes to complete each workout will vary with the individual more than any of the other workouts will. Because there are no base intervals, the swimmer's pace affects the duration. On average, though, the shortest workouts should take about 30 minutes, with the longest at or just under an hour. Before starting these workouts, you should buy a log book if you don't have one already. Logging pool sessions from the beginning will make your progress that much more noticeable and encouraging.

# Fitness 1

Distance: 600 yards

**Warm-Up (ES 1-2)** **150 yards**

6 × 25 easy freestyle with 15 seconds rest

**Kick Set (ES 4-5)** **100 yards**

Using a board and fins
2 × 50 freestyle with 20 seconds rest

2 × 25 freestyle with 10 seconds rest to loosen arms back up (ES 1-2) **50 yards**

**Main Set (ES 4-7)** **225 yards**

1 × 25 freestyle with 20 seconds rest (ES 4)
1 × 75 freestyle with 20 seconds rest (ES 7)
1 × 25 freestyle with 20 seconds rest (ES 4)
1 × 50 freestyle with 20 seconds rest (ES 7)
1 × 25 freestyle with 20 seconds rest (ES 4)
1 × 25 freestyle with 20 seconds rest (ES 7)

**Cool-Down (ES 1)** **75 yards**

3 × 25 easy freestyle with 20 seconds rest

## INSIDE THE WORKOUT

Enjoy the speed of the kick set using a board and fins. This will help you develop the muscles and endurance needed in future kick sets without fins. After holding on to the board while kicking, your arms might be a little stiff, so use the 2 × 25 easy freestyle that follows to get them loose again. The goal of this main set is to still feel strong at the last 25. Use the easy 25s as a breather, and focus on keeping your stroke together as you get tired. Don't worry about speed; focus on completing the set and getting your heart rate up to about 85 percent on the ES 7 swims.

## Fitness                                                          2

Distance: 600 yards

### Warm-Up (ES 1-2)                                      **100 yards**

2 × 50 easy freestyle with 15 seconds rest

### Drill Set (ES 3)                                        **150 yards**

2 × 75 with 20 seconds rest
   First 25—Freestyle One-Arm Drill (right arm)
   Second 25—Freestyle One-Arm Drill (left arm)
   Third 25—freestyle swim, focusing on technique from previous drill

### Main Set (ES 6-7)                                      **250 yards**

1 × 25 freestyle with 20 seconds rest
1 × 50 freestyle with 20 seconds rest
1 × 75 freestyle with 20 seconds rest
1 × 100 freestyle with 20 seconds rest

### Cool-Down (ES 1)                                       **100 yards**

4 × 25 easy freestyle with 20 seconds rest

### INSIDE THE WORKOUT

The drill set is a continuation of the warm-up, so take the drills easy. No need
to push through them or the straight swim, in which the focus should be on the
technique drilled in the first two 25s. The main set is called a ladder set because
it climbs up in distance. (Some longer ladder sets later in the book will also climb
back down in distance.) Focus on maintaining a pace at ES 6 or ES 7 throughout
the four swims so that you still have enough energy to get through the 100 at the
end. Your stroke should stay nice and stretched out, with your heart rate increasing
as the distance of the set increases.

# Fitness      3

Distance: 600 yards

**Warm-Up (ES 1-2)**          **150 yards**

2 × 75 easy freestyle with 20 seconds rest

**Drill Set (ES 3-4)**          **150 yards**

6 × 25 with 15 seconds rest
    #1—Freestyle Hip-Shoulder-Forehead Drill
    #2—freestyle swim, focusing on technique from previous drill
    #3—Freestyle Fist Drill
    #4—freestyle swim, focusing on technique from previous drill
    #5—Freestyle 3-3-3 Drill
    #6—freestyle swim, focusing on technique from previous drill

**Main Set (ES 4-7)**          **200 yards**

4 × 50 with 10 seconds rest
    #1—freestyle (ES 4)
    #2—freestyle (ES 5)
    #3—freestyle (ES 6)
    #4—freestyle (ES 7)

**Cool-Down (ES 1)**          **100 yards**

100 easy freestyle

## INSIDE THE WORKOUT

The drill set incorporates three drills to reinforce the elements of a proper stroke. Use the alternating swims to focus on the emphasized technique from the preceding drill. The main set is based on the principle of descending, which means getting faster with each swim. However, the descending swims are based on effort instead of time. The main goal, besides finishing the entire set, is to gain an understanding of the feeling of getting faster throughout the set as fatigue increases. The time of rest is somewhat minimal to get your heart rate up as the set wears on. It's a short set, though, so if you're feeling good on the last 50, challenge yourself by increasing your tempo to get your effort level up to an 8.

# Fitness 4

Distance: 1,000 yards

### Warm-Up (ES 1-2)                                    **200 yards**

8 × 25 easy freestyle with 15 seconds rest

### Kick Set (ES 4-5)                                   **150 yards**

Using a board and fins
1 × 50 freestyle with 15 seconds rest
1 × 25 freestyle with 10 seconds rest
*Repeat 2 times*

50 easy freestyle to loosen arms back up (ES 1-2)       **50 yards**

### Main Set (ES 1)                                     **450 yards**

6 × 75 with 20 seconds rest
   #1—freestyle (ES 5)
   #2—freestyle (ES 6)
   #3—freestyle (ES 7)
   *Repeat 2 times*

### Cool-Down (ES 1)                                    **150 yards**

3 × 50 easy freestyle with 15 seconds rest

### INSIDE THE WORKOUT

This main set is similar to that in workout 3, but there's more rest between swims to allow a little more time to catch your breath. Because of this luxury, you should be able to focus more on descending each 75 and really feeling the difference between an ES 5 and an ES 7 effort. This is a great set to practice reading the pace clock and recording the times of each swim in your log book. As you flip back through your log in later weeks, you might be amazed at how quickly you've progressed!

# Fitness 5

Distance: 1,000 yards

## Warm-Up/Drill Set (ES 1-3) · 500 yards

4 × 25 easy freestyle with 15 seconds rest (ES 1-2)
3 × 50 easy freestyle with 20 seconds rest (ES 1-2)
2 × 75 drills with 25 seconds rest (ES 3)
  First 25—Freestyle One-Arm Drill (right arm)
  Second 25—Freestyle One-Arm Drill (left arm)
  Third 25—Freestyle 3-3-3 Drill
1 × 100 easy freestyle, focusing on techniques from previous drills

## Main Set (ES 7) · 400 yards

4 × 100 freestyle with 30 seconds rest

## Cool-Down (ES 1) · 100 yards

2 × 50 easy freestyle with 15 seconds rest

## INSIDE THE WORKOUT

The warm-up and drilling have been combined so you can work on stroke technique without fighting fatigue. The main set is pretty straightforward: Keep an ES 7 pace throughout, ensuring that your time for the first 100 is the same as for the fourth. This set will definitely test your swim fitness, but the 30 seconds rest between each 100 will help lower your heart rate and give you a chance to maintain a steady pace.

## Fitness                                                          6

Distance: 1,000 yards

### Warm-Up (ES 1-2)                                          **200 yards**
4 × 50 easy freestyle with 20 seconds rest

### Pull Set (ES 5)                                          **150 yards**
Using a pull buoy and paddles
2 × 75 freestyle with 20 seconds rest

50 easy freestyle (ES 1-2)                                   **50 yards**

### Main Set (ES 7)                                          **500 yards**
1 × 100 freestyle with 15 seconds rest
1 × 75 freestyle with 15 seconds rest
1 × 50 freestyle with 15 seconds rest
1 × 25 freestyle with 15 seconds rest
*Repeat 2 times*

### Cool-Down (ES 1)                                         **100 yards**
4 × 25 easy freestyle with 10 seconds rest

## INSIDE THE WORKOUT

The hard part about this main set is the beginning, with the 100 followed by the 75. Because there isn't a lot of rest between each swim, begin the set relatively slowly so you're not worn out by the time you reach the 25. After all, you do have to repeat this set, while maintaining an ES 7 throughout. This challenging set will really help build your endurance.

# Fitness 7

Distance: 1,500 yards

**Warm-Up (ES 1-2)**                                      **200 yards**

200 easy freestyle

**Kick Set (ES 5)**                                       **200 yards**

Using a board
8 × 25 stroke of your choice with 20 seconds rest

2 × 50 easy freestyle with 15 seconds rest (ES 1-2)      **100 yards**

**Main Set (ES 4-7)**                                     **600 yards**

1 × 25 freestyle with 10 seconds rest (ES 4)
1 × 75 freestyle with 20 seconds rest (ES 7)
*Repeat 6 times*

**Pull Set (ES 5)**                                       **300 yards**

Using a pull buoy and paddles
3 × 100 freestyle with 20 seconds rest, long and stretched out

**Cool-Down (ES 1)**                                      **100 yards**

4 × 25 easy freestyle with 10 seconds rest

## INSIDE THE WORKOUT

Note on the kick set that you get a choice of strokes to kick, but also note that the set calls for no use of fins. The main set is an introduction to the type of active-rest set you'll find in the workouts in chapter 7. However, 75 percent of this set is done at ES 7, whereas in a true active-rest set, that percentage would be lower. As you tire during the 75s, remember you have 20 seconds rest and an easy 25 to look forward to. But don't expect your heart rate to recover completely during the easy part of the set. With only 10 seconds rest after the 25s, you'll probably be pretty fatigued as the set wears on, so focus on keeping your stroke together toward the end.

# Fitness 8

Distance: 1,500 yards

## Warm-Up (ES 1-2) 300 yards

6 × 50 easy freestyle with 15 seconds rest

## Drill Set (ES 3) 400 yards

16 × 25 with 15 seconds rest
Odd 25s—freestyle drill of your choice
Even 25s—freestyle swim, focusing on technique from previous drill

## Main Set (ES 7) 600 yards

2 × 50 freestyle with 10 seconds rest
2 × 100 freestyle with 20 seconds rest
2 × 150 freestyle with 30 seconds rest

## Cool-Down (ES 1) 200 yards

4 × 50 easy freestyle with 20 seconds rest

## INSIDE THE WORKOUT

This main set is the longest yet in the beginner's workout when you consider total distance and length of each swim. If you need to take the effort level down to an ES 6 to get through it, that's okay. There's enough rest on the 100s and 150s to keep you going strong to the end. The way to get through a set like this is to focus on keeping your stroke long and stretched out, even if it feels as if you're carrying a piano on your back! This set is a precursor to some of the Building a Base workouts in the next chapter.

# Fitness 9

Distance: 1,500 yards

## Warm-Up (ES 1-3)        **150 yards**

1 × 75 easy freestyle with 20 seconds rest (ES 1)
1 × 50 easy freestyle with 20 seconds rest (ES 2)
1 × 25 easy freestyle with 20 seconds rest (ES 3)

## Drill Set (ES 4)        **450 yards**

Using fins and paddles
3 × 150 with 30 seconds rest
    First 50—Freestyle Sidekick Drill (25 right arm, 25 left arm)
    Second 50—Freestyle 10-10 Kick Drill
    Third 50—freestyle swim, focusing on techniques from previous drills

## Main Set (ES 7)        **750 yards**

10 × 75 freestyle with 20 seconds rest

## Cool-Down (ES 1)        **150 yards**

150 easy freestyle

## INSIDE THE WORKOUT

The variety in this workout comes in the warm-up (with different lengths of swims and exertion levels) and the kick drill set. The main set is designed simply to practice maintaining a steady pace throughout the 750 yards. The 75s and the set itself are short enough to ensure you can do so. By no means is it easy, but the simplicity of the set should allow you to focus on keeping the same stroke without experiencing too much fatigue toward the end. By now, you should be fit enough that a set like this won't seem intimidating.

# Fitness                                                      10

Distance: 2,000 yards

### Warm-Up (ES 1)                                      600 yards
300 easy freestyle with 30 seconds rest (ES 1)
3 × 100 easy freestyle with 15 seconds rest, working on increasing tempo
(ES 2)

### Pull Set (ES 4-5)                                   300 yards
Using a pull buoy and paddles
6 × 50 freestyle with 15 seconds rest, keeping a steady pace throughout

### Main Set (ES 4-7)                                   750 yards
1 × 50 freestyle with 15 seconds rest (ES 4)
2 × 100 freestyle with 15 seconds rest (ES 7)
*Repeat 3 times*

### Kick Set (ES 5)                                     200 yards
Using a board and fins
4 × 50 freestyle with 20 seconds rest

### Cool-Down (ES 1)                                    150 yards
150 easy freestyle

## INSIDE THE WORKOUT

Try to keep a relatively easy pace throughout the pull set. The challenge of this main set is that there are two 100s in a row at an ES 7 pace. You need to keep the first and second 100s at an even pace to build endurance and increase your ability to swim faster for longer. The 50s are short and don't allow much rest, but they do provide a breather as you become more and more fatigued.

# Fitness 11

Distance: 2,000 yards

## Warm-Up (ES 1-2)      **300 yards**

3 × 100 easy freestyle with 20 seconds rest

## Drill Set (ES 4)      **400 yards**

8 × 50 with 15 seconds rest
    Odd 50s—freestyle drill of your choice
    Even 50s—freestyle swim, focusing on technique from previous drill

## Pre-Main Set (ES 3-6)      **400 yards**

16 × 25 with 10 seconds rest
    #1—freestyle (ES 3)
    #2—freestyle (ES 4)
    #3—freestyle (ES 5)
    #4—freestyle (ES 6)
    *Repeat 4 times*

## Main Set (ES 3-7)      **700 yards**

1 × 25 freestyle with 15 seconds rest (ES 3)
1 × 25 freestyle with 15 seconds rest (ES 7)
1 × 25 freestyle with 15 seconds rest (ES 3)
1 × 50 freestyle with 15 seconds rest (ES 7)
1 × 25 freestyle with 15 seconds rest (ES 3)
1 × 75 freestyle with 15 seconds rest (ES 7)
1 × 25 freestyle with 15 seconds rest (ES 3)
1 × 100 freestyle with 15 seconds rest (ES 7)
*Repeat 2 times*

## Cool-Down (ES 1)      **200 yards**

8 × 25 easy freestyle with 15 seconds rest

## INSIDE THE WORKOUT

The pre-main set is meant to get your heart rate up in preparation for the faster swims in the main set. It's important to build in effort through each round of 4 × 25, with the first and second 25s being relatively easy. But it is just as important to peak at that ES 6 threshold, because the heart of the workout is coming next! The main set looks long and daunting, but it's actually 50 yards shorter than that in workout 10. The goal is to maintain a consistent pace on all of the fast swims. The 15 seconds rest isn't a lot, but the easy 25s offer more down time to give you a physical and mental break before moving on to the next fast swim. The hardest part will be keeping the pace up for the 100 at the end of the set.

## Fitness 12

Distance: 2,000 yards

**Warm-Up (ES 1-2)**     **250 yards**
1 × 250 easy freestyle

**Kick Set (ES 4)**     **300 yards**
Using a board and fins
4 × 75 freestyle with 20 seconds rest

2 × 50 easy freestyle with 15 seconds rest (ES 1-2)     **100 yards**

**Pull Set (ES 5)**     **300 yards**
Using a pull buoy and paddles
4 × 75 freestyle with 20 seconds rest

2 × 50 easy freestyle with 15 seconds rest (ES 1-2)     **100 yards**

**Main Set (ES 4-7)**     **750 yards**
1 × 100 freestyle with 20 seconds rest (ES 4)
3 × 50 freestyle with 20 seconds rest (ES 7)
*Repeat 3 times*

**Cool-Down (ES 1)**     **200 yards**
200 easy freestyle

### INSIDE THE WORKOUT

This group of workouts ends with a classic beginner's active-rest main set. The 100 at ES 4 gives you enough time to recover after the fast 3 × 50s. Again, it's important to swim all 50s at the exact same pace. If you're feeling really good, try to drop your time in the 50s by a second with each set. For example, if you swim :50 on the first three, try to go :49 the second time through and :48 on the third.

# chapter 6

# Building a Base

The 12 workouts in this chapter are intended to help build cardiovascular and muscular endurance. Increasing the ability to swim at a steady rate for extended distances and periods of time improves overall fitness and is an important part of training for competitors. This chapter's workouts prepare the body for the more physically and mentally challenging workouts in chapters to come.

Endurance workouts are distinct from other types in that the overriding training principle is maintaining a steady heart rate throughout the workout. In speed workouts, energy expenditure is in intense bursts at near maximal efforts followed by enough rest to lower the heart rate. But the goal in endurance workouts is to keep the heart rate between 70 and 85 percent of maximum by swimming at a consistent and moderate pace with relatively little rest, especially throughout the main set. Each of these workouts has been written with this principle in mind, and understanding the nuances of how the principle is implemented is valuable for several reasons. First, knowing why each element of a workout is designed the way it is increases the motivation to swim the workout as intended. Although parts of any workout might be challenging, sticking with it is easier if the benefit is understood. Second, if you need to modify a workout for some reason, such as a lack of time one day or lack of equipment, you'll be able to do so while still achieving the most gains possible. Finally, should you want to try your hand at designing workouts, you'll know the concepts that go into effective endurance training.

The intervals in the main sets are on a 1:00 per 50 base. This interval is reasonable but should be altered if necessary to stay within 70 to 85 percent of your maximum heart rate. Kicking, pulling, and drill sets are a bit slower to give swimmers a chance to develop familiarity with the equipment and drills. It is important in these workouts to keep the heart rate steady and not attempt to swim too fast too soon, but it also is essential that swimmers challenge themselves to reap the most rewards from their time in the water.

There should be no rest taken within the set other than that which is built into the base or written into the workout. Extra breaks here and there always feel good, but if the heart rate drops below the optimal zone between repeats, then the workout becomes something other than an endurance workout and no sound training principles are applied. Be sure to take no more than three minutes of rest between sets. Again, too much rest defeats the purpose of steady-state swimming and causes the heart rate to drop below the target window.

Each of these workouts includes a warm-up, a main set, and a cool-down. Each workout also includes at least one additional set such as kicking, pulling, drilling, or sprinting. The steady-swimming principle applies to each part of the workout with the exception of the sprinting sets. To learn to swim faster, you must swim faster. But doing so requires more power than endurance and thus requires the additional rest that's built into those intervals.

The first two workouts are 2,500 yards, and each pair of subsequent workouts increases by 500 yards, with the final two base workouts at 5,000 yards. The shortest workouts should take about 50 minutes to swim, adding about 10 or 12 minutes for every 500-yard increase. Almost all swimming is freestyle.

# Base 1

Distance: 2,500 yards

**Warm-Up (ES 1-2)** **300 yards**

300 easy freestyle, mixing in some backstroke and breaststroke

**Kick Set (ES 4-5)** **200 yards**

Using a board
8 × 25 freestyle on 1:00

50 easy freestyle to loosen arms back up (ES 1-2) **50 yards**

**Pull Set (ES 5-6)** **300 yards**

Using a pull buoy and paddles
4 × 75 freestyle on 1:45

**Main Set (ES 7)** **1,000 yards**

1 × 25 freestyle on :30
1 × 50 freestyle on 1:00
1 × 75 freestyle on 1:30
1 × 100 freestyle on 2:00
*Repeat 4 times*

**Sprint Set (ES 9-10)** **200 yards**

4 × 50 freestyle on 1:30 all-out

**Drill Set (ES 3)** **250 yards**

250 swim
   First 50—Freestyle Hip-Shoulder-Forehead Drill
   Second 50—freestyle swim, focusing on technique from previous drill
   Third 50—Freestyle One-Arm Drill (25 right, 25 left)
   Fourth 50—freestyle swim, focusing on technique from previous drill
   Fifth 50—Freestyle 3-3-3 Drill

**Cool-Down (ES 1)** **200 yards**

200 easy freestyle, mixing in some backstroke and breaststroke

## INSIDE THE WORKOUT

The main set will get harder toward the end of each miniset as the distance increases. There's a bit of a break during the 25s and 50s, but the 75s and 100s will be a challenge. The interval stays the same to keep your heart rate even, so work to maintain a steady pace throughout the set. The sprint set should be swum all-out, so lots of rest has been built in to give your heart rate a chance to return to moderate before you leave the wall for another all-out sprint.

# Base                                                     2

Distance: 2,500 yards

### Warm-Up (ES 1-2)                                      **400 yards**

4 × 100 easy freestyle with 20 seconds rest

### Drill Set (ES 3)                                      **400 yards**

8 × 50 with 10 seconds rest
   Odd 50s—Freestyle Sidekick Drill (25 right arm, 25 left arm)
   Even 50s—Freestyle One-Arm Drill (25 right arm, 25 left arm)

### Pull Set (ES 5-6)                                     **600 yards**

Using a pull buoy and paddles
3 × 200 freestyle on 4:20

### Main Set (ES 7)                                       **900 yards**

3 × 50 freestyle on 1:00
3 × 100 freestyle on 2:00
3 × 150 freestyle on 3:00

### Cool-Down (ES 1)                                      **200 yards**

200 easy freestyle, mixing in some backstroke

## INSIDE THE WORKOUT

The pull set should be swum long and stretched out and at the same pace for each repeat. Be careful not to start out too fast or your shoulders will hurt by the third 200. The main set builds into the distance of the set. Try to keep the same per-50 pace for the entire set, even when the 100s and 150s become more challenging.

# Base                                                            3

Distance: 3,000 yards

## Warm-Up (ES 1-2)                                    **500 yards**
2 × 250 easy freestyle with 30 seconds rest

## Kick Set (ES 4-5)                                   **300 yards**
Using a board
1 × 50 freestyle on 2:00
1 × 25 breaststroke on 1:00
*Repeat 4 times*

100 easy freestyle to loosen arms back up (ES 1-2)    **100 yards**

## Pull Set (ES 5-6)                                   **400 yards**
Using a pull buoy and paddles
400 freestyle, long and stretched out

## Main Set (ES 7)                                   **1,500 yards**
15 × 100
  #s 1-5—freestyle on 2:00
  #s 6-10—freestyle on 1:55
  #s 11-15—freestyle on 1:50

## Cool-Down (ES 1)                                    **200 yards**
200 easy freestyle

## INSIDE THE WORKOUT
The pull set is a straight swim, so make sure to stay long and stretched out. The main set starts out at a moderate 100 base and then decreases five seconds after each set of five. This is challenging because you must get faster throughout the set to make the interval, so conserve energy at the beginning to have enough left to finish strong.

## Base 4

Distance: 3,000 yards

### Warm-Up (ES 1-2)     400 yards
400 easy freestyle, long and stretched out

### Kick Set (ES 4-5)     300 yards
Using a board
6 × 50 on 2:00
    Odd 50s—freestyle
    Even 50s—breaststroke

100 easy freestyle to loosen arms back up (ES 1-2)     100 yards

### Drill Set (ES 3)     300 yards
12 × 25 on :45
    Odd 25s—Freestyle Fist Drill
    Even 25s—freestyle swim, focusing on technique from previous drill

### Main Set (ES 7)     1,750 yards
1 × 250 freestyle on 5:00
2 × 200 freestyle on 4:00
3 × 150 freestyle on 3:00
4 × 100 freestyle on 2:00
5 × 50 freestyle on 1:00

### Cool-Down (ES 1)     150 yards
150 easy freestyle

## INSIDE THE WORKOUT

Use the drill set to feel your forearms moving through the water in a backward-S motion. Focusing on using your hands and forearms will help you swim well through the main set, which is a tough one. Although everything is on the same interval, the distances get shorter, so you're getting less rest between each swim. You'll start to feel the fatigue from the longer distances that lead off the set, so be prepared. Although you think the closing 50s will be a piece of cake, they are actually going to be challenging because you'll probably be pretty tired by the time you get to them.

# Base

Distance: 3,500 yards

**Warm-Up (ES 1-2)**                                    **600 yards**

6 × 100 easy freestyle with 20 seconds rest

**Pull Set (ES 5-6)**                                   **600 yards**

Using a pull buoy and paddles
4 × 150 freestyle on 3:15

**Main Set (ES 7)**                                     **1,800 yards**

6 × 300 freestyle on 6:00, descending #s 1-3 and #s 4-6

**Sprint Set (ES 9-10)**                                **300 yards**

12 × 25 freestyle on :45 all-out!

**Cool-Down (ES 1)**                                    **200 yards**

200 easy freestyle

## INSIDE THE WORKOUT

The main set introduces the concept of descending. Descending a set means starting out on the easy side of moderate and getting faster with each repetition. The descending in this set is broken into two minisets, so you'll descend one to three seconds from the first 300 to the second and then another one to three seconds from the second 300 to the third. You'll then start over with the more moderate base on the fourth 300 and descend the fifth and sixth as you did the second and third. This is difficult to do when you're trying to build a base because you get more tired as the set goes on. Descending forces you to push yourself at the end of the set when you start feeling like you're just going through the motions of getting through the laps. Descending also adds some interest to an otherwise boring set like this one. In the sprint set, remember to swim *all-out*, as fast as you possibly can, for each 25. The 45-second interval should give you enough rest to recover between the 25s, so don't hold back.

# Base 6

Distance: 3,500 yards

**Warm-Up (ES 1-2)**     **600 yards**

600 easy freestyle, long and stretched out

**Kick Set (ES 4-5)**     **450 yards**

Using a board
6 × 75 on 3:00
    Odd 75s—freestyle
    Even 75s—breaststroke

150 easy freestyle to loosen arms back up (ES 1-2)     **150 yards**

**Main Set (ES 7)**     **2,000 yards**

4 × 200 freestyle on 4:00
4 × 150 freestyle on 3:00
4 × 100 freestyle on 2:00
4 × 50 freestyle on 1:00

**Cool-Down (ES 1)**     **300 yards**

300 easy freestyle

## INSIDE THE WORKOUT

The main set starts out with four 200s and four 150s, so expect to be tired by the time you reach the 100s and 50s. You'll need to remain determined to get through this set by keeping everything at an even pace throughout.

# Base                                                      7

Distance: 4,000 yards

## Warm-Up (ES 1-2)                                   **600 yards**
2 × 300 easy freestyle with 20 seconds rest

## Kick Set (ES 4-5)                                  **500 yards**
Using a board and fins
10 × 50 freestyle on 1:15

100 easy freestyle to loosen arms back up (ES 1-2)    **100 yards**

## Pull Set (ES 5-6)                                  **800 yards**
Using a pull buoy and paddles
8 × 100
    #s 1-4—freestyle on 2:10
    #s 5-8—freestyle on 2:05

## Main Set (ES 7)                                    **1,800 yards**
1 × 300 freestyle on 6:00
2 × 150 freestyle on 2:45
*Repeat 3 times*

## Cool-Down (ES 1)                                   **200 yards**
200 easy freestyle

## INSIDE THE WORKOUT

This kick set is the first in this chapter that calls for fins. Enjoy the speed you'll feel using them, but remember to stay focused on your form. The purpose of the main set is to test your endurance. The 300s are on a 1:00 per 50 base, but the 150s are at :55. When you're tired after a long 300, you have to go just as fast or faster on the 150s to make the interval. If the base of 1:00 is somewhat easy for you, challenge yourself to improve by lowering it.

Building a Base

## Base      8

Distance: 4,000 yards

### Warm-Up (ES 1-2)      **500 yards**
500 easy freestyle

### Drill Set (ES 3)      **600 yards**
6 × 100 with 20 seconds rest
    Odd 100s—Freestyle One-Arm Drill (50 right arm, 50 left arm)
    Even 100s—freestyle swim, focusing on technique from previous drill

### Main Set (ES 7)      **2,000 yards**
10 × 200
    #s 1-5—freestyle on 4:00
    #s 6-10—freestyle on 3:50

### Pull Set (ES 5-6)      **600 yards**
Using a pull buoy and paddles
12 × 50 freestyle on 1:10

### Cool-Down (ES 1)      **300 yards**
300 easy freestyle, mixing in some backstroke and breaststroke

### INSIDE THE WORKOUT

This workout is designed to be challenging, so lower the base if you are below 75 percent of your MHR. The main set is another example of testing your endurance as you swim the set. The first five 200s are on a 2:00 per 100 base, with the last five on a 1:55 per 100 base. This means you'll have to work especially hard at the end of the set, even if it feels like your arms are about to fall off! This also helps break up the 2,000 yards. You'll notice the order of the sets in this workout is a little different, with the pulling coming after the main set. That means that even though you worked really hard to hit those intervals in the 200s, you're not quite finished for the day. The good news? The pull set is a moderate 600 yards.

# Base                                                                    9

Distance: 4,500 yards

### Warm-Up (ES 1-2)                                                500 yards
500 easy freestyle

### Kick Set (ES 4-5)                                               300 yards
Using a board
12 × 25 stroke of your choice on 1:00

100 easy freestyle to loosen arms back up (ES 1-2)                 **100 yards**

### Drill Set (ES 3)                                                400 yards
8 × 50 on 1:30
    Odd 50s—Freestyle Hip-Shoulder-Forehead Drill
    Even 50s—freestyle swim, focusing on technique from previous drill

### Pull Set (ES 5-6)                                               600 yards
Using a pull buoy and paddles
1 × 150 freestyle on 3:15
1 × 100 freestyle on 2:10
1 × 50 freestyle on 1:05
*Repeat 2 times*

### Main Set (ES 7)                                               2,500 yards
1 × 100 freestyle on 2:00
1 × 200 freestyle on 4:00
1 × 300 freestyle on 6:00
1 × 400 freestyle on 8:00
1 × 500 freestyle on 10:00
1 × 400 freestyle on 7:40
1 × 300 freestyle on 5:45
1 × 200 freestyle on 3:50
1 × 100 freestyle on 2:00

### Cool-Down (ES 1)                                                100 yards
100 easy freestyle

## INSIDE THE WORKOUT

This main set is a ladder set, climbing up and then back down in distance. Just as with base workouts 7 and 8, the set gets a little faster at the end, so challenge yourself to keep the pace up even when you're tired. In the straight freestyle laps of the drill set, work on the stretching out and rotation motion that is palpable during the Freestyle Hip-Shoulder-Forehead Drill.

# Base 10

Distance: 4,500 yards

## Warm-Up (ES 1-2)                                              800 yards

800 easy freestyle

## Drill Set (ES 3)                                              300 yards

12 × 25 on :45
 #1—Freestyle One-Arm Drill (right arm)
 #2—Freestyle One-Arm Drill (left arm)
 #3—Freestyle 3-3-3 Drill
 #4—freestyle swim, working on techniques from previous drills
 *Repeat 3 times*

## Main Set (ES 7)                                            2,500 yards

5 × 500 freestyle on 10:00, descending #s 1-5

## Sprint Set (ES 2-10)                                         600 yards

2 × 25 freestyle on :45 all-out
1 × 50 freestyle (ES 2)
1 × 50 freestyle on 1:30 all-out (ES 10)
*Repeat 4 times*

## Cool-Down (ES 1)                                             300 yards

300 easy freestyle

## INSIDE THE WORKOUT

This is a classic workout to build your endurance base. Building means more than simply maintaining, and this main set illustrates that distinction with a longer descent than you saw in base 5. Descend by 3 to 5 seconds for each 500 so that there's about a 15- to 20-second difference between the first and last 500s. The first 500 is on the moderate 1:00 per 50 base, and although 5 seconds might sound like a big chunk of time, it's only a quarter of a second per lap when spread out over a 500. Push yourself with a lower base for best results if you can handle it. In the sprint set, the goal is to add the times from your 2 × 25 together and then try to match or beat that speed in your 50. The longer sprint and easy 50 in between gives this sprint set an endurance feel. It's tough, but it helps build what we call "easy speed," which is discussed in the introduction of the next chapter. In the drill set early in the workout, work on the underwater pull that's emphasized in the Freestyle One-Arm Drill and Freestyle 3-3-3 Drill.

# Base                                                                11

Distance: 5,000 yards

### Warm-Up (ES 1-2)                                           **900 yards**
6 × 150 easy freestyle with 10 seconds rest

### Kick Set (ES 4-5)                                          **600 yards**
Using board and fins
2 × 50 freestyle on 1:15 (ES 4)
1 × 100 freestyle on 2:20 (ES 5)
*Repeat 3 times*

100 easy freestyle to loosen arms back up (ES 1-2)            **100 yards**

### Main Set (ES 7)                                         **3,000 yards**
1 × 100 freestyle on 2:00
2 × 200 freestyle on 4:00
3 × 300 freestyle on 6:00
4 × 400 freestyle on 8:00

### Sprint Set (ES 9-10)                                       **200 yards**
8 × 25 on :45 freestyle all-out

### Cool-Down (ES 1)                                           **200 yards**
200 easy freestyle

## INSIDE THE WORKOUT

The challenge in this workout starts early with the kick set. Although you get to use fins, the 100s are longer than the 50s and swum on a faster base. Be prepared for your legs to burn, but push through it for excellent long-term results. The main set is also meant to be tough, so lower that base if you find this set on the easy side. Although the interval doesn't change with the set, you'll probably feel fatigue setting in before you even start the 400s. The key is to go out at a moderate pace on the 100s and 200s so you have something left for the 300s and 400s.

## Base 12

Distance: 5,000 yards

### Warm-Up (ES 1-2) 800 yards

800 easy freestyle, swimming your favorite freestyle drill every fourth 50

### Pull Set (ES 5-6) 900 yards

Using a pull buoy and paddles
12 × 75 freestyle on 1:45

### Main Set (ES 7) 3,000 yards

2 × 500 freestyle on 10:00
5 × 200 freestyle on 3:50
10 × 100 freestyle on 1:50

### Cool-Down (ES 1) 300 yards

300 easy freestyle

### INSIDE THE WORKOUT

The main set is swum on an increasingly faster base as it progresses. At 3,000 yards it is a long set, so there's a real endurance factor involved. Managing your pace throughout the set—fast enough to keep up with the intervals yet not so fast as to hit the wall by the end—is crucial to meeting the challenge. As always, lower that base if you can handle a faster pace for the distance.

# chapter 7

# Increasing Anaerobic Threshold

One of the physiological keys to being able to swim faster for longer is the body's anaerobic threshold, or the absolute maximum level of effort at which the body can continue to transport enough oxygen to and lactic acid from the muscles. It's one thing to be able to swim at ES 2 indefinitely. It's quite another to be able to swim at ES 7 indefinitely. The higher your anaerobic threshold, the less difficult it will feel to go faster. This ease in swimming fast is what swimmers call "easy speed."

Anaerobic threshold workouts are those in which the effort falls in that small window between an aerobic workout, which primarily improves cardiovascular fitness, and an anaerobic workout, which primarily improves raw speed. An endurance workout is considered aerobic because the effort level is such that the body can keep up with the muscles' demand for oxygen for relatively longer periods of time. An anaerobic workout requires such a high level of effort that the body's rate of supplying the muscles with the necessary amount of oxygen is insufficient to sustain the effort for more than about 60 seconds.

These workouts get away from the even pace of the base workouts of chapter 6 and introduce effort levels that vary much more within a set. The training still works on endurance to some extent, but it will feel more like you're working on speed. Incorporating that speed without spending as much time at the wall as you will in the speed workouts trains your body to swim faster for longer.

I consider anaerobic threshold workouts, also called "active rest," to be the most enjoyable. Active rest is the concept of allowing the heart rate to drop (the rest part) while you're swimming (the active part), instead of while you're at the wall. The levels of speed and physical exertion required within a set change often, so workouts never get stale. The faster pace gets the heart rate up to about 90 percent of your maximum, but the slower-paced swims at about 70 percent give you a chance to recover before the next fast swim. These workouts should help you develop or hone your ability to distinguish between varying effort levels.

As in the previous chapter, the workouts start at 2,500 yards, and every other one increases by 500 yards to a maximum of 5,000 yards. The workouts should take about the same amount of time as the base workouts, the shortest at about 50 minutes and increasing by about 10 to 12 minutes with each 500-yard increase. Almost all of the swimming is freestyle.

# Anaerobic Threshold                                   1

Distance: 2,500 yards

## Warm-Up (ES 1-2)                              **400 yards**

4 × 100 easy freestyle with 15 seconds rest

## Drill Set (ES 3-4)                            **300 yards**

6 × 50 on 1:15
   #1—25 Freestyle One-Arm Drill (right arm), 25 freestyle swim
   #2—25 Freestyle One-Arm Drill (left arm), 25 freestyle swim
   #3—25 Freestyle 3-3-3 Drill, 25 freestyle swim
   *Repeat 2 times*

## Pull Set (ES 5-6)                             **400 yards**

Using a pull buoy and paddles
400 freestyle, long and stretched out

## Main Set (ES 4-8)                           **1,200 yards**

1 × 100 freestyle on 2:20 (ES 4)
4 × 75 freestyle on 1:20 (ES 8)
*Repeat 3 times*

## Cool-Down (ES 1)                              **200 yards**

200 easy freestyle

## INSIDE THE WORKOUT

This first anaerobic threshold workout features a classic active-rest main set. The fast 75s are broken up with slower 100s that should allow heart rates to lower a bit. Although you're still swimming, the pace is relatively easy. To increase anaerobic threshold, it's important to maintain speed in the 4 × 75, even if you're getting tired in the middle of them. Keep up the pace. After all, you get to "rest" during the 100s!

## Anaerobic Threshold                                    2

Distance: 2,500 yards

### Warm-Up (ES 1-2)                                   **500 yards**
2 × 250 easy freestyle with 20 seconds rest

### Kick Set (ES 4-5)                                  **600 yards**
Using a board and fins
12 × 50 freestyle on 1:15

### Main Set (ES 4-8)                               **1,200 yards**
1 × 50 freestyle on 1:05 (ES 4)
1 × 100 freestyle on 1:45 (ES 8)
*Repeat 8 times*

### Cool-Down (ES 1)                                   **200 yards**
4 × 50 easy freestyle with 10 seconds rest

### INSIDE THE WORKOUT

This is another classic active-rest set, with the 50s giving heart rates a chance to return to about 70 percent MHR from the 90 percent effort required by the 100s. If you need to swim the 50s on an even slower interval to catch your breath, go ahead.

# Anaerobic Threshold

Distance: 3,000 yards

**Warm-Up (ES 1-2)**            **400 yards**

400 easy freestyle

**Drill Set (ES 3-4)**            **300 yards**

12 × 25 on :45
     #1—Freestyle Hip-Shoulder-Forehead Drill
     #2—freestyle swim, focusing on technique from previous drill
     #3—Freestyle Fist Drill
     #4—freestyle swim, focusing on technique from previous drill
     *Repeat 3 times*

**Main Set (ES 6-8)**            **1,500 yards**

15 × 100
     #1—freestyle on 1:55 (ES 6)
     #2—freestyle on 1:50 (ES 7)
     #3—freestyle on 1:45 (ES 8)
     *Repeat 5 times*

**Pull Set (ES 5-6)**            **600 yards**

Using a pull buoy and paddles
4 × 150 freestyle on 3:15

**Cool-Down (ES 1)**            **200 yards**

2 × 100 easy freestyle with 10 seconds rest

## INSIDE THE WORKOUT

Use the drill set to fine-tune your stroke, concentrating on the technique that each drill emphasizes in the following freestyle swim. The main set is challenging—it's not quite a perfect active-rest set. The ES is slightly different for each 100, which allows the opportunity to learn to pace yourself and recognize the subtle differences in effort level required. Obviously, there is no easy swimming in this set; the intervals get more difficult with each trio of 100s. This is the kind of set that develops easy speed.

## Anaerobic Threshold                                    4

Distance: 3,000 yards

### Warm-Up (ES 1-2)                                     **600 yards**

3 × 200 easy freestyle with 20 seconds rest

### Drill Set (ES 4-5)                                   **750 yards**

10 × 75 with 10 seconds rest
    First 25—Freestyle Sidekick Drill (right arm)
    Second 25—Freestyle Sidekick Drill (left arm)
    Third 25—Backstroke 10-10 Kick Drill

### Main Set (ES 4-8)                                   **1,500 yards**

2 × 75 freestyle on 1:40 (ES 4)
1 × 150 freestyle on 2:40 (ES 8)
*Repeat 5 times*

### Cool-Down (ES 1)                                     **150 yards**

150 easy freestyle

### INSIDE THE WORKOUT

The kicking drills get you good and warm before the main set, which is a great active-rest set because 50 percent of the distance is swum at ES 4. This doesn't mean you're taking the day off from work, though. The set is designed to rest you in preparation for the 150s so you can maintain a fast pace for those laps.

Increasing Anaerobic Threshold

# Anaerobic Threshold                                            5

Distance: 3,500 yards

### Warm-Up (ES 1-2)                                    **600 yards**
600 easy freestyle, mixing in some backstroke, breaststroke, and drills

### Pull Set (ES 5-6)                                   **800 yards**
Using a pull buoy and paddles
4 × 200 freestyle on 4:20

### Main Set (ES 6-8)                                 **1,800 yards**
1 × 300 freestyle on 5:45 (ES 6)
1 × 200 freestyle on 3:40 (ES 7)
1 × 100 freestyle on 1:45 (ES 8)
*Repeat 3 times*

### Cool-Down (ES 1)                                    **300 yards**
3 × 100 easy freestyle with 10 seconds rest

### INSIDE THE WORKOUT

This main set is a longer active-rest set because of the 300s. The key is keeping the 300s long and stretched out while maintaining a good pace. The descending interval—the base per 100 gets five seconds faster with each repeat—will definitely prove challenging, and you'll have to demonstrate some endurance to repeat the miniset three times.

# Anaerobic Threshold                                            6

Distance: 3,500 yards

## Warm-Up (ES 1-2)                                    **600 yards**

8 × 75 easy freestyle with 10 seconds rest

## Kick Set (ES 4-5)                                   **600 yards**

Using a board
12 × 50 on 1:45
    Odd 50s—freestyle
    Even 50s—butterfly or breaststroke

200 easy freestyle to loosen arms back up (ES 1-2)     **200 yards**

## Main Set (ES 4-8)                                 **1,800 yards**

2 × 150 freestyle on 2:50 (ES 8)
1 × 200 freestyle on 4:20 (ES 4)
2 × 150 freestyle on 2:45 (ES 8)
1 × 200 freestyle on 4:20 (ES 4)
2 × 150 freestyle on 2:40 (ES 8)
1 × 200 freestyle on 4:20 (ES 4)
2 × 150 freestyle on 2:35 (ES 8)

## Cool-Down (ES 1)                                    **300 yards**

12 × 25 easy freestyle with 5 seconds rest

## INSIDE THE WORKOUT

Notice that the 150s in the main set have a descending time interval but stay at an ES 8. The goal is to maintain a consistent pace on those 150s throughout the set, resulting in less and less rest before the 200s as the set progresses. Endurance really comes into play in the second half of the set. The secret is to use the 200s to recover in preparation for the 150s.

# Anaerobic Threshold

Distance: 4,000 yards

### Warm-Up (ES 1-3)         **600 yards**

6 × 100 freestyle with 15 seconds rest
    #s 1-2—easy freestyle (ES 1)
    #s 3-4—easy freestyle (ES 2)
    #s 5-6—easy freestyle (ES 3)

### Drill Set (ES 3-4)         **600 yards**

2 × 25 with 10 seconds rest—Freestyle Hip-Shoulder-Forehead Drill
1 × 50 with 10 seconds rest—freestyle swim, focusing on technique
       from previous drill
*Repeat 6 times*

### Pull Set (ES 5-6)         **600 yards**

Using a pull buoy and paddles
2 × 300 freestyle with 20 seconds rest, long and stretched out

### Main Set (ES 4-8)         **2,000 yards**

1 × 200 freestyle on 4:20 (ES 4)
6 × 50 freestyle on :55 (ES 8)
*Repeat 4 times*

### Cool-Down (ES 1)         **200 yards**

200 easy freestyle, mixing in some backstroke, breaststroke, and drills

## INSIDE THE WORKOUT

Half of the total distance in the drill set is straight swimming. Use those laps to focus on the hand position on entry into the water and the angle of the body throughout the swim. The main set incorporates more speed because of the relatively short distance of the ES 8 repetitions. This allows you to focus on swimming fast during the 50s, which certainly isn't easy but does allow for a bit more rest than some of the other sets that include 150s or 200s.

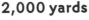

Increasing Anaerobic Threshold

Distance: 4,000 yards

### Warm-Up (ES 1-2) **500 yards**
500 easy freestyle, mixing in some freestyle drills
20 seconds rest

### Pull Set (ES 5) **500 yards**
Using a pull buoy and paddles
500 freestyle

100 easy freestyle (ES 1-2) **100 yards**

### Drill Set (ES 4) **600 yards**
Using fins and paddles
4 × 150 on 3:15
   First 50—Freestyle One-Arm Drill (25 right arm, 25 left arm)
   Second 50—Freestyle 3-3-3 Drill
   Third 50—freestyle swim, working on increasing tempo

100 easy freestyle **100 yards**

### Main Set (ES 4-8) **2,000 yards**
1 × 100 freestyle on 2:10 (ES 4)
1 × 100 freestyle on 1:45 (ES 8)
1 × 100 freestyle on 2:10 (ES 4)
2 × 100 freestyle on 1:45 (ES 8)
1 × 100 freestyle on 2:10 (ES 4)
3 × 100 freestyle on 1:45 (ES 8)
1 × 100 freestyle on 2:10 (ES 4)
4 × 100 freestyle on 1:45 (ES 8)
1 × 100 freestyle on 2:10 (ES 4)
5 × 100 freestyle on 1:45 (ES 8)

### Cool-Down (ES 1) **200 yards**
200 easy freestyle

### INSIDE THE WORKOUT

Each group of 100s at ES 8 should be treated as its own miniset, with the easy 100s between the time to recover and the time to start preparing for the next group of 100s. Once again, starting out at a strong pace that doesn't seem like too much of a sprint helps to maintain that pace throughout the set. That's all you have to do—maintain—because the ES 8 intervals don't get faster as the set wears on. Just make sure to use the easy 100s to rest.

Distance: 4,500 yards

## Warm-Up (ES 1-2)     **600 yards**

4 × 50 easy freestyle with 10 seconds rest
2 × 100 easy freestyle with 15 seconds rest
1 × 200 easy freestyle with 20 seconds rest

## Kick Set (ES 4-10)     **600 yards**

Using a board
24 × 25 on :55
    #1—breaststroke or butterfly (ES 4-5)
    #s 2-3—freestyle sprint (ES 9-10)
    *Repeat 8 times*

200 easy freestyle to loosen arms back up (ES 1-2)     **200 yards**

## Main Set (ES 4-8)     **1,950 yards**

1 × 100 freestyle on 2:15 (ES 4)
2 × 150 freestyle on 2:40 (ES 8)
1 × 100 freestyle on 2:15 (ES 4)
4 × 100 freestyle on 1:45 (ES 8)
1 × 100 freestyle on 2:15 (ES 4)
6 × 75 freestyle on 1:20 (ES 8)
1 × 100 freestyle on 2:15 (ES 4)
8 × 50 freestyle on :55 (ES 8)

## Drill Set (ES 3-4)     **400 yards**

4 × 100 with 15 seconds rest
    First 50—freestyle drill of your choice
    Second 50—freestyle swim, focusing on technique from previous drill

## Pull Set (ES 5-6)     **600 yards**

Using a pull buoy and paddles
12 × 50
    #1—freestyle on 1:05
    #2—freestyle on 1:00
    #3—freestyle on :55
    #4—freestyle on :50
    *Repeat 3 times*

*Increasing Anaerobic Threshold*

*(continued)*

**Cool-Down (ES 1)** 150 yards

3 × 50 easy freestyle with 10 seconds rest

### INSIDE THE WORKOUT

This main set is another that requires learning to pace yourself to get through it. The distances of each group of fast swims decrease, but the number of repetitions increases. All are within a couple of seconds of the same base. Between it all, though, are only 400 yards at ES 4, so both endurance and easy speed are needed to push through this set. The drill and pull sets following the main set incorporate more endurance into the workout, especially the pulling, which is descending.

Distance: 4,500 yards

**Warm-Up (ES 1-3)**                                    **900 yards**

4 × 100 easy freestyle on 2:20 (ES 1)
6 × 50 easy freestyle on 1:10 (ES 2)
8 × 25 easy freestyle on :35 (ES 3)

**Pull Set (ES 5-6)**                                   **1,000 yards**

Using a pull buoy and paddles
1 × 100 freestyle on 2:10
1 × 200 freestyle on 4:20
1 × 300 freestyle on 6:30
1 × 400 freestyle on 7:40

100 easy freestyle (ES 1-2)                             **100 yards**

**Main Set (ES 4-8)**                                   **2,000 yards**

1 × 50 freestyle on 1:10 (ES 4)
1 × 200 freestyle on 3:30 (ES 8)
1 × 100 freestyle on 2:15 (ES 4)
1 × 150 freestyle on 2:40 (ES 8)
1 × 150 freestyle on 3:20 (ES 4)
1 × 100 freestyle on 1:45 (ES 8)
1 × 200 freestyle on 4:25 (ES 4)
1 × 50 freestyle on :50 (ES 8)
*Repeat 2 times*

**Sprint Set (ES 3-9)**                                 **300 yards**

12 × 25 on :45
    Odd 25s—freestyle (ES 3)
    Even 25s—freestyle (ES 9)

**Cool-Down (ES 1)**                                    **200 yards**

200 easy freestyle

**INSIDE THE WORKOUT**

The swims in the pull set get longer, so use that as a reminder to keep your stroke long and stretched out as well. Even though the main set seems long, half of it is relatively easy. It is a great active-rest set because you can build into a really fast 50 by the end of it. If you can go especially fast toward the end of the set, this will really help your easy speed.

Increasing Anaerobic Threshold

Distance: 5,000 yards

**Warm-Up (ES 1-3)** 900 yards

9 × 100 with 15 seconds rest
 #s 1-3—easy freestyle (ES 1)
 #s 4-6—easy freestyle (ES 2)
 #s 7-9—easy freestyle (ES 3)

**Drill Set (ES 3-4)** 500 yards

10 × 50 on 1:15
 Odd 50s—freestyle drill of your choice
 Even 50s—freestyle swim, focusing on technique from previous drill

**Main Set (ES 4-8)** 2,400 yards

12 × 200
 Odd 200s—freestyle on 4:30 (ES 4)
 Even 200s—freestyle on 3:30 (ES 7-8)

**Pull Set (ES 5-6)** 900 yards

Using a pull buoy and paddles
3 × 150 freestyle on 3:15
3 × 100 freestyle on 2:10
3 × 50 freestyle on 1:05

**Cool-Down (ES 1)** 300 yards

6 × 50 easy freestyle with 15 seconds rest

**INSIDE THE WORKOUT**

You have freedom in this workout to swim your favorite drills. Just remember to focus on that technique during the straight swim. The main set is uncomplicated—12 × 200. The easy 200s are a full minute slower that the fast 200s, so take advantage of the easy ones to prepare for the fast ones. The challenge will be to keep the same pace on all six fast 200s, so this set will likely test your endurance.

Increasing Anaerobic Threshold

# Anaerobic Threshold                                    12

Distance: 5,000 yards

**Warm-Up (ES 1-2)**                                    **800 yards**

2 × 400 easy freestyle, starting out easy and building slightly

**Drill Set (ES 5)**                                    **600 yards**

Using fins
4 × 150 with 20 seconds rest
    First 50—Butterfly Inverted Kick Drill
    Second 50—backstroke kick in streamline position
    Third 50—Freestyle Sidekick Drill (25 right arm, 25 left arm)

100 easy freestyle to loosen arms back up (ES 1-2)     **100 yards**

**Pull Set (ES 5-6)**                                   **1,000 yards**

Using a pull buoy and paddles
5 × 200 on 4:20 freestyle, keeping a steady pace throughout

100 easy freestyle (ES 1-2)                             **100 yards**

**Main Set (ES 4-8)**                                   **2,250 yards**

1 × 150 freestyle on 3:15 (ES 4)
3 × 100 freestyle on 1:45 (ES 8)
*Repeat 5 times*

**Cool-Down (ES 1)**                                    **150 yards**

150 easy freestyle

## INSIDE THE WORKOUT

The drill set calls for the use of fins, so enjoy the speed! Then focus on keeping an even pace on all five 200 pulls. This group of workouts ends with another classic active-rest set. By now you should know what to do; especially important is using those easy 150s to recover.

# chapter 8

# Increasing Speed

Sprint workouts have an entirely different feel to them than any other type of swim workout. The distances swum are shorter, the rest between swims is longer, and the intensity of each swim is higher. The intent of a sprint workout is clear and simple: to train the body to swim at top speed. Just as you must train the body to swim farther (in endurance workouts) or to swim faster for longer (in anaerobic threshold workouts), you must also train the body to swim with speed.

Muscle memory is more important than many swimmers realize. No one doubts the process of learning a certain skill—such as shooting a basketball or throwing a football—through practicing that skill over and over. Less obvious is the need to teach the body what it feels likes to move fast through the water, how to maintain coordination and perform the technique accurately at a high rate of speed and to supply energy to the muscles more efficiently.

Sprint workouts do that by changing the patterns of rest and effort level. The amount of rest built into each interval is significantly longer—often more than twice the time—than intervals in other workouts. But those breaks come at a price, and that price is an exertion level that is all-out or almost all-out for much of the main set.

The effort levels in an aerobic workout are low enough to enable the body to deliver the muscles a continual supply of oxygen. The effort levels of a sprint workout are so high that the muscles use oxygen at a faster rate than the body can replenish it. The muscles rely instead on the body's anaerobic energy system. Continuing at a high exertion level requires giving the body time to almost fully recover before sprinting again; otherwise the workout becomes a tiring aerobic set in which huge amounts of effort are put out to sustain a relatively slow pace.

The key to getting the most out of sprint workouts is following the set exactly as it is written. If a set calls for a swim at ES 9 or ES 10, that's what it means! That is the effort level at which the body will learn to swim faster. Equally important is to take all of the recommended rest. You need to get your heart rate completely down before you start the next all-out swim. If you feel yourself tightening up while you're resting on the wall, slowly swim half a length down and back to stay loose. Some of the main sets include some active rest, and others are simply all-out sprints with lots of rest.

Warm-ups and cool-downs are particularly important in sprint workouts. You are taxing your muscles to the max, and you need to take good care of them. Some of the workouts include pre-main sets designed to get your heart rate up a bit and make it easier to go into full-sprint mode. One or two swim sets incorporate the use of fins and paddles. These basically continue the warm-up to get your heart rate and tempo up and ensure you're ready for the main set. Sets with fins and paddles also allow you to experience what fast swimming feels like. Even though the muscles are being aided in swimming faster, they are developing the muscle memory that is necessary to eventually swim faster without the gear.

The workouts in this chapter cover less total distance, but they are not shorter, and by no means are they easier. They are grouped by threes instead of by twos, starting at 1,500 yards and building to 3,000 yards. However, they take as long or longer than the base or AT (anaerobic threshold) workouts because of the rest between swims.

# Sprint 1

Distance: 1,500 yards

## Warm-Up (ES 1-2)       400 yards
4 × 100 easy freestyle with 20 seconds rest

## Drill Set (ES 3-4)       300 yards
4 × 75 on 2:00
   First 25—Freestyle One-Arm Drill (right arm)
   Second 25—Freestyle One-Arm Drill (left arm)
   Third 25—freestyle swim, focusing on technique from previous drill

## Main Set (ES 8-10)       600 yards
12 × 50 on 2:15, descending #s 1-3
   #1—freestyle (ES 8)
   #2—freestyle (ES 9)
   #3—freestyle (ES 10)
   *Repeat 4 times*

## Cool-Down (ES 1)       200 yards
200 easy freestyle

### INSIDE THE WORKOUT
The main set in this first sprint workout incorporates descending, so each 50 should be swum a little faster than the previous one. The first 50 of each miniset is on a really easy 2:15, so you should be getting a little more than a minute of rest between each. Even though the ES 8s are easier than the ES 9s and ES 10s, they are still pretty fast and require you to get your heart rate up.

Increasing Speed

# Sprint                                                                 2

Distance: 1,500 yards

## Warm-Up (ES 1-2)                                          **300 yards**
300 easy freestyle

## Drill Set (ES 4-5)                                        **300 yards**
Using fins and paddles
6 × 50 on 1:30
    #1—Freestyle Sidekick Drill (right arm)
    #2—Freestyle Sidekick Drill (left arm)
    #3—freestyle swim, focusing on technique from previous drill
    *Repeat 2 times*

100 easy freestyle                                           **100 yards**

## Main Set (ES 9)                                           **600 yards**
1 × 75 freestyle on 3:15
1 × 50 freestyle on 2:15
1 × 25 freestyle on 2:15
*Repeat 4 times*

## Cool-Down (ES 1)                                          **200 yards**
2 × 100 easy freestyle with 15 seconds rest, mixing in some backstroke and breaststroke

## INSIDE THE WORKOUT
Work on getting your turnover up during the laps of straight swimming in the drill set. This will help your speed later in the workout—and in future swims. The intervals for the 50 and the 25 are the same; this is to allow plenty of rest after the 25 to prepare for the 75 sprint. There's no active rest in this set—no easy laps—so every swim is almost an all-out sprint. Every swim in this set must be at close to the same speed. The natural tendency will be to back off your pace on the 75s and 50s, but keep your focus and use the extra time after the 25s to catch your breath for the 75s. This will significantly help your speed in the future!

Increasing Speed

# Sprint                                                   3

Distance: 1,500 yards

## Warm-Up (ES 1-2)                                **400 yards**

8 × 50 easy freestyle with 10 seconds rest, working on increasing tempo

## Pull Set (ES 5)                                 **300 yards**

Using a pull buoy and paddles
2 × 150 freestyle with 20 seconds rest, long and stretched out

100 easy freestyle (ES 1-2)                        **100 yards**

## Main Set (ES 3-9)                               **500 yards**

20 × 25 on 1:15
   #1—freestyle (ES 3)
   #s 2-4—freestyle (ES 9)
   *Repeat 5 times*

## Cool-Down (ES 1)                                **200 yards**

2 × 100 easy freestyle with 15 seconds rest, mixing in some backstroke and breaststroke

## INSIDE THE WORKOUT

Use the warm-up to start preparing your body for the sprints that follow by increasing your tempo slightly with each 50. The main set might remind you of an active-rest workout, but the massive amounts of rest make it more of a sprint session. The set consists of only 25s, which is everyone's favorite distance in a sprint workout. They are much less daunting and exhausting than all-out 50s or 100s. Ideally, you should be getting about a minute of rest after each of the 25s at ES 9. The key is to keep the last fast 25s at the same speed or faster than the first fast 25s each time through.

Increasing Speed

# Sprint 4

Distance: 2,000 yards

## Warm-Up (ES 1-2)                                                     500 yards

1 × 100 easy freestyle with 20 seconds rest
1 × 75 easy freestyle with 15 seconds rest
1 × 50 easy freestyle with 10 seconds rest
1 × 25 easy freestyle with 5 seconds rest
*Repeat 2 times*

## Fins and Paddles Set (ES 5-6)                                        600 yards

6 × 100 with 15 seconds rest
   #s 1-2—freestyle, long and stretched out (ES 5)
   #s 3-4—freestyle with paddles, long and stretched out (ES 6)
   #s 5-6—freestyle with paddles and fins, working on a fast tempo (ES 6)

100 easy freestyle (ES 1-2)                                            100 yards

## Main Set (ES 3-9)                                                    600 yards

6 × 25 freestyle on 1:10 (ES 9)
1 × 50 freestyle on 2:00 (ES 3)
4 × 50 freestyle on 2:15 (ES 9)
1 × 50 freestyle on 2:00 (ES 3)
2 × 75 freestyle on 3:20 (ES 9)

## Cool-Down (ES 1)                                                     200 yards

8 × 25 easy freestyle with 10 seconds rest

## INSIDE THE WORKOUT

The fins and paddles set gives your muscles a chance to swim faster than you can without the aid of gear. Experiencing speed is an important part of getting faster—and it's fun! The main set, though, is pretty tough. At the height of it (the 4 × 50) is 200 yards of really fast swimming with no easy yards in between. The 50s will probably tire you, but the real challenge comes with the 75s that follow. Not only are they longer, but they come at the end of the set. There's not much leeway in how fast you swim at an ES 9 pace, so concentrate on using the significant amounts of rest and the easy 50s to get your heart rate down, and think of how much faster you'll be because of the hard work.

Increasing Speed

# Sprint                                                    5

Distance: 2,000 yards

## Warm-Up (ES 1-2)                                      **500 yards**
500 easy freestyle

## Kick Set (ES 4)                                       **300 yards**
Using a board
4 × 75 freestyle on 2:15

100 easy freestyle to loosen arms back up (ES 1-2)        **100 yards**

## Pull Set (ES 5)                                       **300 yards**
Using a pull buoy and paddles
4 × 75 freestyle on 2:00

## Main Set (ES 8-10)                                    **600 yards**
6 × 100 on 4:30, descending #s 1-3
   #1—freestyle (ES 8)
   #2—freestyle (ES 9)
   #3—freestyle (ES 10)
   *Repeat 2 times*

## Cool-Down (ES 1)                                      **200 yards**
200 easy freestyle, mixing in some backstroke

## INSIDE THE WORKOUT
This main set is another in which each swim should be a few seconds faster than the previous. Use the pace clock to check your time after each swim. This is a true sprint set with ample rest, but it will be challenging because 100s are hard to swim at such a fast pace. You should take at least three minutes of rest between each 100, so adjust intervals as necessary. If you feel yourself tightening up while resting on the wall, swim a few easy strokes.

Increasing Speed

Distance: 2,000 yards

### Warm-Up (ES 1-2)     **500 yards**

5 × 100 easy freestyle with 15 seconds rest, working on increasing tempo

### Drill Set (ES 3)     **450 yards**

9 × 50 on 1:30
   #1—25 Freestyle Fist Drill, 25 freestyle swim
   #2—25 Freestyle Hip-Shoulder-Forehead Drill, 25 freestyle swim
   #3—25 Freestyle 3-3-3 Drill, 25 freestyle swim
   *Repeat 3 times*

### Main Set (ES 3-9)     **800 yards**

1 × 100 freestyle on 4:30 (ES 9)
100 freestyle on 4:00 (ES 3)
2 × 75 freestyle on 3:20 (ES 9)
100 freestyle on 4:00 (ES 3)
3 × 50 freestyle on 2:15 (ES 9)
100 freestyle on 4:00 (ES 3)
4 × 25 freestyle on 1:10 (ES 9)

### Cool-Down (ES 1)     **250 yards**

250 easy freestyle

### INSIDE THE WORKOUT

In the warm-up, build with each 100 so that by the fourth lap you have a good tempo. The main set might be a bit deceiving. The 1 × 100 and 2 × 75 might seem like the most difficult part of the set, but fatigue will sneak up on you during the 3 × 50. Use the "gimme" 100s at ES 3 to get your heart rate back down, and then enjoy the fast 25s to close out the set.

Increasing Speed

Distance: 2,500 yards

### Warm-Up (ES 1-2)                                    **500 yards**
2 × 250 easy freestyle with 30 seconds rest, followed immediately by pull set

### Pull Set (ES 5)                                     **500 yards**
Using a pull buoy and paddles
2 × 250 freestyle with 30 seconds rest, long and stretched out

### Pre-Main Set (ES 4-7)                               **200 yards**
8 × 25 on :55
   #1—freestyle (ES 4)
   #2—freestyle (ES 5)
   #3—freestyle (ES 6)
   #4—freestyle (ES 7)
   *Repeat 2 times*

### Main Set (ES 3-10)                                  **750 yards**
1 × 50 freestyle on 2:15 (ES 8)
1 × 25 freestyle on 1:10 (ES 10)
1 × 50 freestyle on 2:00 (ES 3)
*Repeat 6 times*

### Drill Set (ES 3-4)                                  **300 yards**
12 × 25 on :55
   Odd 25s—freestyle drill of your choice
   Even 25s—freestyle swim, focusing on technique from previous drill

### Cool-Down (ES 1)                                    **250 yards**
5 × 50 easy freestyle with 10 seconds rest

## INSIDE THE WORKOUT

This workout features several sets designed to slowly raise and then lower your heart rate. The pre-main set should be used to work on getting your tempo up as the ES increases. That build-up, combined with the 50s at ES 8 in the main set, will prime you for the all-out 25s that are the focus of the workout. The 50s are at a fast pace, but the 25s are at a rare ES 10, so rise to the challenge and give each your best effort, although the 50s will likely cause some fatigue. The easy 50s are a chance to prepare physically and mentally for the next round of the set.

Increasing Speed

# Sprint 8

Distance: 2,500 yards

| | |
|---|---|
| **Warm-Up (ES 1-2)** | **600 yards** |

3 × 200 easy freestyle with 20 seconds rest

| | |
|---|---|
| **Drill Set (ES 4)** | **600 yards** |

Using fins
4 × 150 with 15 seconds rest
    First 50—Freestyle Sidekick Drill (right arm)
    Second 50—backstroke kick in streamline position
    Third 50—Freestyle Sidekick Drill (left arm)

| | |
|---|---|
| 100 easy freestyle (ES 1-2) | **100 yards** |

| | |
|---|---|
| **Main Set (ES 6-10)** | **750 yards** |

10 × 75 on 3:20
    #1—freestyle (ES 6)
    #2—freestyle (ES 7 )
    #3—freestyle (ES 8)
    #4—freestyle (ES 9)
    #5—freestyle (ES 10)
    *Repeat 2 times*

| | |
|---|---|
| **Pull Set (ES 4-5)** | **300 yards** |

Using a pull buoy and paddles
300 freestyle, long and stretched out

| | |
|---|---|
| **Cool-Down (ES 1)** | **150 yards** |

150 easy freestyle

## INSIDE THE WORKOUT

The main set includes some active rest, but it's heavier on the active than the rest compared to anaerobic threshold workouts. After swimming five increasingly fast 75s, climaxing at near maximum and then maximum effort, you roll right into a 75 at ES 6—slower, of course, but still classified as a significant effort. You'll have to rely on your fitness on the first two 75s at ES 6 and ES 7 to get your heart rate close to normal before sprinting again on the last three. The 3:20 interval is generous, though, which allows time to recover.

Increasing Speed

# Sprint 9

Distance: 2,500 yards

### Warm-Up (ES 1-2)                                        **500 yards**

500 easy freestyle

### Pull Set (ES 5)                                         **600 yards**

Using a pull buoy and paddles
1 × 300 freestyle with 30 seconds rest
1 × 200 freestyle with 20 seconds rest
1 × 100 freestyle with 10 seconds rest

### Pre-Main Set (ES 4-7)                                   **400 yards**

4 × 100 on 2:30
   #1—freestyle (ES 4)
   #2—freestyle (ES 5)
   #3—freestyle (ES 6)
   #4—freestyle (ES 7)

### Main Set (ES 3-10)                                      **800 yards**

4 × 50 freestyle on 1:45 (ES 7)
100 freestyle on 2:45 (ES 3)
3 × 50 freestyle on 1:45 (ES 8)
100 freestyle on 2:45 (ES 3)
2 × 50 freestyle on 1:45 (ES 9)
100 freestyle on 2:45 (ES 3)
1 × 50 freestyle on 1:45 (ES 10)

### Cool-Down (ES 1)                                        **200 yards**

2 × 100 easy freestyle with 15 seconds rest

## INSIDE THE WORKOUT

This is another workout that builds throughout, and it includes swims at every ES level. Increase your tempo as the pull set progresses to get ready for the sprints. Then use the pre-main set to build in intensity to ES 7, which is where the main set starts. The points of emphasis of the main set are the 2 × 50 at ES 9 and the 1 × 50 at ES 10, but you can't ignore that the set of 4 × 50 and 3 × 50 need to be swum at a pretty good clip as well. This is primarily a sprint set, but the first seven 50s will test your endurance also.

Increasing Speed

Distance: 3,000 yards

## Warm-Up (ES 1-3)                                                600 yards

1 × 150 easy freestyle with 20 seconds rest (ES 1)
1 × 100 easy freestyle with 15 seconds rest (ES 2)
1 × 50 easy freestyle with 10 seconds rest (ES 3)
*Repeat 2 times*

## Drill Set (ES 3-4)                                               600 yards

8 × 75 with 15 seconds rest
First 25—Freestyle One-Arm Drill (right arm)
Second 25—Freestyle One-Arm Drill (left arm)
Third 25—freestyle swim, focusing on technique from previous drill

## Fins and Paddles Set (ES 4-6)                                    600 yards

12 × 50 on 1:15
#1—freestyle (ES 4)
#2—freestyle (ES 5)
#3—freestyle (ES 6)
*Repeat 4 times*

## Main Set (ES 3-10)                                             1,000 yards

40 × 25 on 1:00
1 × 25—easy freestyle (ES 3)
5 × 25—fast freestyle (ES 9-10)
1 × 25—easy freestyle (ES 3)
4 × 25—fast freestyle (ES 9-10)
1 × 25—easy freestyle (ES 3)
3 × 25—fast freestyle (ES 9-10)
1 × 25—easy freestyle (ES 3)
2 × 25—fast freestyle (ES 9-10)
1 × 25—easy freestyle (ES 3)
1 × 25—fast freestyle (ES 9-10)
*Repeat 2 times*

## Cool-Down (ES 1)                                                 200 yards

200 easy freestyle, mixing in backstroke, breaststroke, butterfly, and drills

Increasing Speed

## INSIDE THE WORKOUT

As in previous workouts, increase your tempo as you increase in effort level throughout the fins and paddles set. Then enjoy this ultimate sprint set! Everyone loves 25s, and you get plenty of them in this workout. Feel free to swim the first two groups of 25s (5 × 25 and 4 × 25) at an ES 9 and then build into an ES 10 pace as the repeats get shorter. You'll get plenty of rest on the wall and enough active rest with the easy 25s to keep you fresh for each batch of fast 25s.

Increasing Speed

Distance: 3,000 yards

| **Warm-Up (ES 1-2)** | **600 yards** |

4 × 150 easy freestyle with 15 seconds rest

| **Kick Set (ES 4-5)** | **400 yards** |

Using a board
8 × 50 freestyle on 2:00, descending #s 1-4 and #s 5-8

| 100 easy freestyle to loosen arms back up (ES 1-2) | **100 yards** |

| **Main Set (ES 3-9)** | **1,200 yards** |

2 × 50 freestyle on 2:00 (ES 8)
1 × 100 freestyle on 4:00 (ES 3)
1 × 100 freestyle on 4:00 (ES 9)
*Repeat 4 times*

| **Pull Set (ES 5)** | **500 yards** |

Using a pull buoy and paddles
500 freestyle, long and stretched out

| **Cool-Down (ES 1)** | **200 yards** |

4 × 50 easy freestyle with 15 seconds rest

## INSIDE THE WORKOUT

The descend in this workout appears in the kick set, with two rounds of descending 50s. The primary points of emphasis of the main set are the fast 100s at ES 9, but that doesn't mean you can slack off on the 50s. ES 8 is still a very serious effort. Focus on your tempo and easy speed during the 50s, and use that feeling to make your 100s even faster. The added recovery time during the easy 100s will help.

Increasing Speed

# Sprint 12

Distance: 3,000 yards

**Warm-Up (ES 1-2)** **600 yards**

2 × 300 easy freestyle with 30 seconds rest

**Drill Set (ES 3-4)** **400 yards**

16 × 25 with 10 seconds rest
    Odd 25s—freestyle drill of your choice
    Even 25s—freestyle swim, focusing on technique from previous drill

**Pre-Main Set (ES 3-7)** **500 yards**

10 × 50 on 1:15
    #1—freestyle (ES 3)
    #2—freestyle (ES 4)
    #3—freestyle (ES 5)
    #4—freestyle (ES 6)
    #5—freestyle (ES 7)
    *Repeat 2 times*

100 easy freestyle (ES 1-2) **100 yards**

**Main Set (ES 3-10)** **800 yards**

8 × 100 on 4:30
    #1—freestyle (ES 3)
    #2—freestyle (ES 10)
    *Repeat 4 times*

**Pull Set (ES 5)** **400 yards**

Using a pull buoy and paddles
8 × 50 freestyle with 15 seconds rest, long and stretched out

**Cool-Down (ES 1)** **200 yards**

200 easy freestyle

## INSIDE THE WORKOUT

Use the 25s of straight swimming in the drill set to hone your technique, and then build throughout the pre-main set in preparation to swim all-out. Although the main set might look daunting because of the 100s at ES 10, think about it in more manageable terms. It is only 800 yards, and half of that is at an easy ES 3. That leaves only 400 hard yards, so really attack them. Swim *all-out* for the entire 100, and welcome the challenge!

Increasing Speed

# chapter 9

# Swimming the IM

Variety adds spice to this chapter of workouts, where you'll find a little bit of everything—kicking, pulling, drilling, sprinting, and swimming the freestyle, backstroke, breaststroke, and butterfly. Depending on your choice of drills in a couple of workouts, you might swim all four strokes in every workout, so turn to this chapter to keep your sessions in the pool fresh and motivating.

An individual medley (IM) is a race in which one swimmer swims all four strokes an equal distance in a specific order—butterfly, backstroke, breaststroke, and freestyle. The strokes are arranged strategically, starting with the stroke commonly deemed the hardest (butterfly) and followed by the easier backstroke. The difficulty increases again with the breaststroke, and the most familiar stroke—the freestyle—wraps the medley up. In official meets, the IM is swum in three distances: the 100, 200, and 400.

The workouts in this chapter are designed to help swimmers build up to complete a set of 200 IMs by the last workout. To do these workouts, swimmers need a good knowledge of how to swim all four strokes, although the butterfly will be swum the least. Because IM workouts are more endurance based than speed based, they are excellent for aerobic conditioning.

IM workouts can be very fatiguing, so these are calculated a little differently from workouts in other chapters. The time intervals are slower, and there are more rest intervals than are found in all but the chapter on fitness. Not many swimmers have mastered all four strokes, especially fitness swimmers. Some strokes will come more naturally than others for each swimmer. For the best balance of challenge and enjoyment of these workouts, modify the base for one or more of the strokes or drills so that your heart rate stays within 70 to 85 percent MHR range.

The amount of rest between repeats and sets is the same as for the base workouts in chapter 6. However, because the intervals are slower, the IM workouts take longer than others of the same distance. The workout distances again come in pairs, starting at 2,500 and increasing by 500 yards until they reach 5,000 yards.

Pulling is not emphasized in this chapter. It is impossible to pull butterfly, and pulling breaststroke is rare. Backstroke and freestyle pulling will be incorporated periodically. Backstroke pulling can be difficult for beginners, but it does help the underwater stroke. The best kind of IM workout is simply swimming IMs! The workouts are tough physically, but they fly by because there's always something different coming up next.

# Individual Medley                                                    1

Distance: 2,500 yards

### Warm-Up (ES 1-2)                                          **400 yards**
400 easy freestyle, swimming backstroke or breaststroke every fourth 25

### Kick Set (ES 5)                                           **450 yards**
Using a board
6 × 75 breaststroke on 3:15

50 easy freestyle to loosen arms back up (ES 1-2)             **50 yards**

### Main Set (ES 7)                                         **1,000 yards**
1 × 25 on :45 freestyle
1 × 50 on 1:45 (25 breaststroke, 25 freestyle)
1 × 75 on 2:45 (25 backstroke, 25 breaststroke, 25 freestyle)
1 × 100 on 3:45 (25 butterfly, 25 backstroke, 25 breaststroke, 25 freestyle)
*Repeat 4 times*

### Drill Set (ES 3)                                          **400 yards**
8 × 50 on 1:50
    #1—25 Butterfly 3-3-3 Drill, 25 butterfly swim
    #2—25 Backstroke 3-3-3 Drill, 25 backstroke swim
    #3—25 breaststroke pull with freestyle kick, 25 breaststroke swim
    #4—25 Freestyle 3-3-3 Drill, 25 freestyle swim
    *Repeat 2 times*

### Cool-Down (ES 1)                                          **200 yards**
200 easy freestyle, mixing in some backstroke and breaststroke

## INSIDE THE WORKOUT

The concept of a ladder workout is applied to this main set to introduce the individual medley. The main set starts with a 25 of the last stroke that is swum in an official IM race—the freestyle. Each subsequent repetition adds a 25 of the next previous stroke in the IM until the 100 is made up of butterfly, backstroke, breaststroke, and freestyle 25s. This set is a great starter IM workout because it involves only four laps of butterfly, which for many swimmers is the most difficult stroke in terms of both execution and fatigue. The drill set comes late in the workout and allows for practice of each stroke.

Swimming the IM

# Individual Medley

Distance: 2,500 yards

## Warm-Up (ES 1-2)                                    400 yards

16 × 25 easy with 10 seconds rest
  Odd 25s—freestyle
  Even 25s—backstroke

## Drill Set (ES 4)                                    450 yards

9 × 50 on 2:00
  #1—Backstroke Sidekick Drill (25 right arm, 25 left arm)
  #2—Freestyle Sidekick Drill (25 right arm, 25 left arm)
  #3—Breaststroke Heels-to-Fingertips Drill (25),
      Breaststroke Up-Out-Together Drill (25)
  *Repeat 3 times*

## Main Set (ES 5-7)                                   1,500 yards

1 × 100 freestyle on 2:00 (ES 5-6)
1 × 50 butterfly on 1:15 (ES 7)
1 × 50 backstroke on 1:15 (ES 7)
1 × 50 breaststroke on 1:30 (ES 7)
*Repeat 6 times*

## Cool-Down (ES 1)                                    150 yards

150 easy freestyle

## INSIDE THE WORKOUT

The kick set and the drill set are combined in this workout to provide an opportunity to work on the technique of each stroke's kick before swimming the main set, in which the emphasis is on butterfly, backstroke, and breaststroke 50s. The freestyle 100s are on a slow interval and allow a chance to catch your breath. Adjust the intervals according to your abilities in each stroke, but make sure the 100s are fairly easy.

Swimming the IM

# Individual Medley                                              3

Distance: 3,000 yards

**Warm-Up (ES 1-2)**                                    **400 yards**

4 × 100 easy freestyle with 15 seconds rest

**Drill Set (ES 3-4)**                                  **300 yards**

12 × 25
    Odd 25s—freestyle swim on :45
    Even 25s—backstroke, breaststroke, or butterfly drill of your choice on :55

**Main Set (ES 7)**                                     **1,500 yards**

20 × 75 on 2:35
    First 25—backstroke
    Second 25—breaststroke
    Third 25—freestyle

**Pull Set (ES 5)**                                     **600 yards**

Using a pull buoy and paddles
4 × 150 with 15 seconds rest
    First 50—freestyle
    Second 50—backstroke
    Third 50—freestyle

**Cool-Down (ES 1)**                                    **200 yards**

200 easy freestyle

## INSIDE THE WORKOUT

You might notice the warm-up in this workout includes only the freestyle. The drill set that follows provides ample opportunity to warm up the other strokes before the main set. If you're following the workouts in order, you've already done a 100 IM four times within a main set in IM workout 1. Essentially, this main set is full of 100 IMs minus the butterfly lap. Taking out the butterfly here should make the set easy enough for you to make the interval while building your stamina and confidence to do a full set of 100 IM repeats in the not-too-distant future. Keeping an even pace through the entire set is important in building that base.

*Swimming the IM*

## Individual Medley                                              4

Distance: 3,000 yards

### Warm-Up (ES 1-2)                                    **600 yards**
600 swim
  100 easy freestyle
  50 easy backstroke
  100 easy freestyle
  50 easy breaststroke
  *Repeat 2 times*

### Kick Set (ES 4)                                     **600 yards**
Using a board and fins
8 × 75 on 2:30
  Odd 75s—freestyle
  Even 75s—butterfly

100 easy freestyle to loosen arms back up (ES 1-2)     **100 yards**

### Main Set (ES 7)                                   **1,500 yards**
10 × 150 on 4:30
  25—backstroke
  50—breaststroke
  75—freestyle

### Cool-Down (ES 1)                                    **200 yards**
200 easy freestyle, mixing in some backstroke and breaststroke

### INSIDE THE WORKOUT

The kick set in this workout should be fun because you use fins for the flutter and dolphin kicks. The main set helps build up to full IM repeats. Swimming 150s might seem somewhat daunting at first, but look at it more closely. The butterfly has been omitted, and 50 percent of the set is freestyle, which allows a break before swimming the backstroke and breaststroke again. This should make the workout easier if you're relatively new to IM work.

Swimming the IM

# Individual Medley                                          5

Distance: 3,500 yards

### Warm-Up (ES 1-2)                                    **500 yards**
500 easy freestyle

### Drill Set (ES 3-4)                                  **600 yards**
8 × 75 on 3:00
   First 25—Butterfly 3-3-3 Drill
   Second 25—Backstroke 3-3-3 Drill
   Third 25—Breaststroke 3-2-1 Drill

### Main Set (ES 7)                                     **1,800 yards**
12 × 100
   Odd 100s on 2:00—freestyle
   Even 100s on 2:45—backstroke

1-minute rest

12 × 50
   Odd 50s on 1:00—freestyle
   Even 50s on 1:30—breaststroke

### Sprint Set (ES 8-9)                                 **400 yards**
16 × 25 on 1:00
   #1—freestyle (ES 2-3)
   #2—butterfly (ES 8-9)
   #3—freestyle (ES 2-3)
   #4—backstroke (ES 8-9)
   #5—freestyle (ES 2-3)
   #6—breaststroke (ES 8-9)
   #7—freestyle (ES 2-3)
   #8—freestyle (ES 8-9)
   *Repeat 2 times*

### Cool-Down (ES 1)                                    **200 yards**
200 easy freestyle

## INSIDE THE WORKOUT

The freestyle 100s and 50s are meant to be easier than the backstroke and breaststroke swims. Adjust the time standards so you get no more than 10 seconds of rest after each 100 and 7 to 8 seconds of rest after each 50. Enjoy building your speed on the nonfreestyle strokes while getting enough rest to go all-out for each sprint.

Distance: 3,500 yards

### Warm-Up (ES 1-2)                                  **600 yards**

3 × 200 easy freestyle with 20 seconds rest, mixing in some backstroke
and breaststroke

### Kick Set (ES 4-5)                                 **400 yards**

Using a board
8 × 50 breaststroke on 2:10

100 easy freestyle to loosen arms back up (ES 1-2)    **100 yards**

### Main Set (ES 7)                                   **1,600 yards**

1 × 25 butterfly on :55
1 × 25 backstroke on :55
1 × 25 breaststroke on :55
1 × 25 freestyle on :55
1 × 100 IM on 3:45
*Repeat 8 times*

### Pull Set (ES 4-5)                                 **600 yards**

Using a pull buoy and paddles
4 × 150 on 3:30 freestyle

### Cool-Down (ES 1)                                  **200 yards**

200 easy freestyle

## INSIDE THE WORKOUT

Use the kicking set to really work on the up-out-together motion of the breaststroke kick, making sure to kick your ankles all the way together. This is a tough main set for a couple of reasons. One, it's not sprinkled with freestyle to break up the other strokes. Two, it doesn't skimp on the butterfly. That double whammy, though, is countered by fairly slow intervals to provide you with a good amount of recovery time. Feel free to take up to 15 to 20 seconds of rest after each IM, so factor that in as you prepare to use the pace clock in the next intervals. This set is the first in which the IM strokes are swum in order throughout, which is important to the goal of building up to a 200 IM. Afterward, it will feel good just to stretch out with a nice, relaxed freestyle pulling set.

Swimming the IM

Distance: 4,000 yards

**Warm-Up (ES 1-2)**                                                                  **600 yards**

6 × 100 easy freestyle with 15 seconds rest, swimming breaststroke
      or backstroke the last 25 of each 100

**Drill Set (ES 3-4)**                                                                **600 yards**

24 × 25 with 10 seconds rest
    #1—Butterfly Inverted Kick Drill
    #2—Backstroke Sidekick Drill (alternating arms)
    #3—Breaststroke Heels-to-Fingertips Drill
    #4—Freestyle Sidekick Drill (alternating arms)
    *Repeat 6 times*

100 easy freestyle                                                                   **100 yards**

**Pull Set (ES 5-6)**                                                                **600 yards**

Using a pull buoy and paddles
12 × 50
    #s 1-2—freestyle on 1:15
    #3—backstroke on 1:30
    *Repeat 4 times*

100 easy freestyle (ES 1-2)                                                          **100 yards**

**Main Set (ES 5-7)**                                                              **1,800 yards**

1 × 150 freestyle on 3:00 (ES 5-6)
1 × 75 backstroke on 2:00 (ES 7)
1 × 75 breaststroke on 2:15 (ES 7)
*Repeat 6 times*

**Cool-Down (ES 1)**                                                                 **200 yards**

200 easy freestyle, mixing in some backstroke and breaststroke

## INSIDE THE WORKOUT

This workout includes a set that combines kicking and drilling. Concentrate on staying in the streamline position during the butterfly, backstroke, and freestyle kicking drills, and focus on the motion of the legs during all four strokes. The main set is another that emphasizes the backstroke and breaststroke. Like the main set in IM workout 2, the freestyle 150s should be swum at a long, stretched-out pace, with the backstroke and breaststroke 75s being the challenging part of the set. This is the last set in this workout, so don't hold back.

Swimming the IM

## Individual Medley 8

Distance: 4,000 yards

### Warm-Up (ES 1-2)     **750 yards**

3 × 250 easy freestyle with 30 seconds rest, mixing in some backstroke
     and breaststroke

### Drill Set (ES 3-4)     **750 yards**

10 × 75 with 15 seconds rest
  Odd 75s
    First 25—Freestyle One-Arm Drill (right arm)
    Second 25—Freestyle One-Arm Drill (left arm)
    Third 25—freestyle swim, focusing on technique from previous drill
  Even 75s
    First 25—Backstroke One-Arm Drill (right arm)
    Second 25—Backstroke One-Arm Drill (left arm)
    Third 25—backstroke swim, focusing on technique from previous drill

100 easy freestyle     **100 yards**

### Main Set (ES 5-7)     **2,100 yards**

1 × 50—freestyle on 1:15 (ES 5)
1 × 50—freestyle on 1:00 (ES 7)
1 × 50—freestyle on 1:15 (ES 5)
1 × 100—50 breaststroke, 50 freestyle on 2:15 (ES 7)
1 × 50—freestyle on 1:15 (ES 5)
1 × 150—50 backstroke, 50 breaststroke, 50 freestyle on 3:30 (ES 7)
1 × 50—freestyle on 1:15 (ES 5)
1 × 200—IM on 4:30 (ES 7)
*Repeat 3 times*

### Cool-Down (ES 1)     **300 yards**

300 easy freestyle

### INSIDE THE WORKOUT

This drill set is full of single-arm drills and is all about the upper body after the previous workout's kicking and drilling set. Focus on the proper motion and path each arm makes in the freestyle and backstroke. The main set is an introduction to a 200 IM, which is a perfect IM distance for swimmers because of the great fitness benefits derived. However, jumping from a 100 IM to a 200 IM can be overwhelming. So, similar to IM workout 1 in which you gradually built into a 100 IM, this set gently builds into a 200 IM. The intervals for every freestyle in this set are slow and intended to be an easy recovery between the other swims.

# Individual Medley 9

Distance: 4,500 yards

## Warm-Up (ES 1-2)     **800 yards**

16 × 50 with 10 seconds rest
   Odd 50s—easy freestyle
   Even 50s—easy backstroke or breaststroke

## Kick Set (ES 4)     **600 yards**

Using fins
6 × 100 with 20 seconds rest
   #s 1-2—freestyle with board
   #s 3-4—butterfly with board
   #s 5-6—backstroke in streamline position, no board

100 easy freestyle to loosen arms back up (ES 1-2)     **100 yards**

## Drill Set (ES 3-4)     **400 yards**

16 × 25 with 15 seconds rest
   #1—Butterfly One-Arm Drill (your choice of arm)
   #2—butterfly swim
   #3—Backstroke One-Arm Drill (your choice of arm)
   #4—backstroke swim
   #5—Breaststroke 3-2-1 Drill
   #6—breaststroke swim
   #7—Freestyle One-Arm Drill (your choice of arm)
   #8—freestyle swim
   *Repeat 2 times*

100 easy freestyle (ES 1-2)     **100 yards**

## Main Set (ES 5-7)     **2,000 yards**

20 × 100
   Odd 100s—freestyle on 2:15 (ES 5)
   Even 100s—IM on 2:30 (ES 7)

## Sprint Set (ES 9)     **200 yards**

8 × 25 IM order on 1:00 all-out
   #1—butterfly
   #2—backstroke
   #3—breaststroke
   #4—freestyle
   *Repeat 2 times*

*(continued)*

Swimming the IM

### Cool-Down (ES 1)        **300 yards**

4 × 75 easy freestyle with 15 seconds rest

### INSIDE THE WORKOUT

This main set is similar to the one in IM workout 6. This main set is longer but shouldn't be seen as harder. The freestyle 100s should be easy, and the intervals on the IM 100s should be comfortable, with about 10 to 15 seconds of rest after each. Essentially, this is an active-rest IM set, focusing on getting through a 100 IM comfortably. It also will continue to give you confidence as you build into the very difficult sets of multiple 200 IMs in a row. Remember to sprint almost all-out through the two rounds of 25s in IM order (butterfly, backstroke, breaststroke, freestyle).

Swimming the IM

# Individual Medley 10

Distance: 4,500 yards

## Warm-Up (ES 1-2) 1,000 yards

400 easy freestyle with 30 seconds rest, swimming backstroke
   or breaststroke every fourth lap
300 easy freestyle with 20 seconds rest, swimming backstroke
   or breaststroke every third lap
200 easy freestyle with 10 seconds rest, swimming backstroke
   or breaststroke every even lap
100 easy freestyle, mixing in some backstroke and breaststroke

## Pull Set (ES 4-5) 600 yards

Using a pull buoy and paddles
600 freestyle, long and stretched out

100 easy freestyle (ES 1-2) **100 yards**

## Drill Set (ES 3-4) 600 yards

12 × 50 with 20 seconds rest
 #1—butterfly drill of your choice
 #2—backstroke drill of your choice
 #3—breaststroke drill of your choice
 #4—freestyle drill of your choice
 *Repeat 3 times*

100 easy freestyle (ES 1-2) **100 yards**

## Main Set (ES 7) 1,800 yards

12 × 150 on 5:10
 First 50—backstroke
 Second 50—breaststroke
 Third 50—freestyle

## Cool-Down (ES 1) 300 yards

300 easy freestyle

## INSIDE THE WORKOUT

In this workout we're working toward a 200 IM. This set is meant to be a distance IM set to build endurance. The interval is only a suggestion. Alter it as needed so that the most rest you get between repeats is 15 seconds. That is not a lot of time to catch your breath after swimming three different strokes for this distance, but get through this set of 150s and you'll have the confidence you need to complete a 200 IM.

# Individual Medley

Distance: 5,000 yards

## Warm-Up (ES 1-2)                                          1,200 yards
2 × 600 with 30 seconds rest
  First 600—easy freestyle
  Second 600—easy, mixing strokes and drills

## Drill Set (ES 3-4)                                          750 yards
10 × 75 with 15 seconds rest
  First 25—Butterfly Inverted Kick Drill
  Second 25—Backstroke Sidekick Drill
  Third 25—Breaststroke Up-Out-Together Drill

150 easy freestyle to loosen arms back up (ES 1-2)            **150 yards**

## Main Set (ES 3-7)                                        2,000 yards
1 × 100 freestyle on 2:00 (ES 3)
1 × 100 IM on 2:15 (ES 6)
1 × 100 freestyle on 2:00 (ES 3)
1 × 200 IM on 4:30 (ES 7)
*Repeat 4 times*

## Pull Set (ES 4)                                            600 yards
Using a pull buoy and paddles
3 × 200 freestyle with 30 seconds rest, long and stretched out

## Cool-Down (ES 1)                                           300 yards
6 × 50 easy freestyle with 20 seconds rest

## INSIDE THE WORKOUT
We've finally come to our 200 IM! Use the 100 IM in the main set to build into the feeling of swimming all four strokes and the easy 100 freestyle to catch your breath before swimming an entire 200 IM. You'll have another easy 100 to catch your breath before starting over again. The easy freestyle swimming should break the set up enough to make it doable for most proficient IM swimmers. Note the difference in ES between the 100 and 200 IMs, and relish your accomplishment afterward.

Swimming the IM

# Individual Medley    12

Distance: 5,000 yards

## Warm-Up (ES 1-2)                                   1,200 yards

8 × 150 with 20 seconds rest
  First 50—easy freestyle
  Second 50—easy, stroke of your choice
  Third 50—easy freestyle

## Drill Set (ES 3-4)                                 1,200 yards

10 seconds rest between each swim
1 × 50 Butterfly 3-3-3 Drill
1 × 25 butterfly swim
1 × 50 Backstroke 3-3-3 Drill
1 × 25 backstroke swim
1 × 50 Breaststroke 3-2-1 Drill
1 × 25 breaststroke swim
1 × 50 Freestyle 3-3-3 Drill
1 × 25 freestyle swim
*Repeat 4 times*

## Main Set (ES 3-8)                                  1,800 yards

1 × 50 on 1:00 butterfly (ES 7)
1 × 50 on 1:00 backstroke (ES 7)
1 × 50 on 1:10 breaststroke (ES 7)
1 × 50 on 1:00 freestyle (ES 7)
1 × 100 on 2:00 freestyle (ES 3)
1 × 200 on 4:10 IM (ES 8)
1 × 100 on 2:00 freestyle (ES 3)
*Repeat 3 times*

## Pull Set (ES 5)                                    500 yards

Using a pull buoy and paddles
500 freestyle, long and stretched out

## Cool-Down (ES 1)                                   300 yards

3 × 100 easy freestyle with 20 seconds rest

Swimming the IM

*(continued)*

**INSIDE THE WORKOUT**

This main set features three "broken" 200 IMs (because you'll be taking a break after each stroke) and three full 200 IMs. For the advanced swimmer, the goal should be to add up your times in the 4 × 50s—the broken 200 IM—and try to beat that time in the full 200 IM. This is very challenging because, obviously, you're not getting any rest between the 50s during the full swim. Make sure to get at least 10 seconds of rest between each of the ES 7 swims and at least 20 seconds of rest after the 200 IM. The 500 pull will feel good after such a hard IM set. Keep your heart rate fairly low on this nice, long swim.

Swimming the IM

# part III

# The Programs

The essentials of swimming covered in part I were brought to life in the workouts in part II. Now it's time to put those 60 workouts into a more meaningful context. In the same way that engaging workouts enhance the enjoyment factor of swimming, the arrangement of workouts into programs can instill purpose into your training routine and promote your progress as a swimmer.

A well-designed program that fits your ability, goals, and available training time provides two factors that are key to a swimmer's development: consistency and structure. Both keep the body on a steady and focused progression to maximize fitness and improvement. A relatively constant, steady regimen is much more effective than an inconsistent schedule in which the number of times you get to the pool vacillates each week or month. Swimmers retain their confidence and all-important feel for the water with regular pool time. The actual arrangement of the regularly scheduled workouts also is of consequence. Randomly choosing a workout from this book each day before you head to the pool is not a poor method for gaining fitness. But by understanding and following the key principles that characterize a properly designed program, your rate of improvement should increase significantly.

The 12 programs in chapter 10 vary greatly in difficulty, which ensures that at least one is an appropriate starting point for almost any swimmer. The programs are also progressive in a few ways. The average total distance of the workouts gradually increases, as does the number of workouts in a week and the number of weeks in the program. They are designed to help you progress through the programs at your own pace, or to have several programs from which to choose if your schedule fluctuates such that the amount of time you have in a day or week decreases or increases.

The programs are designed to increase your fitness and swimming performance, but they aren't designed to prepare you for a specific race. The intricacies and individuality of training for competition are such that designing a one-size-fits-all program, in fact, would truly fit only one swimmer, if that. Details such as the specific race distance and stroke, ability level, time available, past training programs, and tapering are vital to developing a personalized program that gets you physically and mentally ready for competition. Chapter 11 explains how to train for a race, including the phases of swim training and, most specifically, the tapering process. It also describes the value of rest and cross-training to your overall competitiveness and explains how to determine when and how much of a break to take from intense training. By applying the guidelines to your time frame and situation, your chances of success will increase significantly.

# chapter 10

# Levels 1-6

Welcome to the programs! Used properly, this chapter should lead you to better physical, mental, and emotional health and fitness. Your work in getting to this point—gathering equipment; studying technique; understanding swim training; and perhaps practicing drills, starting your core exercise routine, and testing the workouts—has been well worth your time. You're now ready to take the next step toward improvement as a swimmer.

The 12 programs in this chapter provide you with 72 weeks—more than a year's worth—of swimming plans. They also serve as examples of how to put together your own program if you want to vary your routine. The programs are divided into six levels, with two in each level. Each program pulls workouts from the five chapters in part II, and the average distance of the workouts in the programs gradually increases with each successive level. The programs are based on our four guiding principles:

**1. Variety.** Each program includes all five types of workouts: building swim fitness, building a base, increasing anaerobic threshold, increasing speed, and swimming the IM. Only at levels 4 through 6 are workouts infrequently repeated within a program. The order of the types of workouts also varies each week.

**2. Hard–easy.** Hard workouts are followed either by a day off or a relatively easy workout. For instance, a base workout is followed by a fitness or anaerobic threshold workout to give you a chance to stretch out the sore muscles that might have developed from the base workout the day before. Individual medley workouts are usually followed by fitness workouts for the same reason. In general, sprint workouts don't cause much soreness, so those are added for a change of pace.

**3. Progression.** The programs progress in total distance and intensity. The workouts in each program are based on a certain distance—level 1 on 2,500 yards, level 2 on 3,000, level 3 on 3,500, level 4 on 4,000, level 5 on 4,500, and level 6 on 5,000. But by no means are those distances the only ones swum at each level. For instance, fitness and speed workouts are comparatively shorter than the others, and the latter half of each program includes at least one workout at a longer distance to begin preparing those who are striving to move up to the next level. The programs also increase in number of weeks as the total distance per workout increases because it takes the body longer to adapt to the extra distances.

**4. Spacing.** The workouts are spaced as evenly as possible over each week of the program. Swimming three days a week should mean you never have to swim two days in a row, although your schedule might dictate otherwise now and then. A four-workout week means swimming on consecutive days at least once, and a five-workout week requires swimming consecutive days at least twice. The best swim program, though, will minimize those instances. Swimming three straight days and taking off four is much less effective than swimming two straight days only once a week.

When set up according to these principles, programs can be altered or created to fit anyone's schedule, goals, or ability while still providing a great training regimen. Not every athlete who swims three times a week can get to the pool every Monday, Wednesday, and Friday, as the three-days-a-week programs are written (which is a good thing because pools would be very crowded on these days!). Even if you can follow the programs to a T the majority of the time, life will inevitably cause disruption now and then. Job, family, sickness, injury, vacations, or other commitments might force you to adjust your swimming routine. When that happens, don't despair, and definitely don't stop swimming. Simply adjust the programs to fit your needs by moving the workouts to your available swimming days, keeping in mind the four principles we've discussed.

The programs in this book can be used in several ways. Some swimmers might choose one program and follow it indefinitely. This develops a great fitness base, but because the body adapts to exercise and requires higher intensity levels to make greater fitness gains, this plan might not allow them to reach their full potential. Other swimmers might choose to swim both the A and B programs at a level before moving up to the next level. This approach requires flexibility in the number of times they get to the pool in a given period, but it offers the easiest way to progress through the programs. Some swimmers might choose to continue following either the A or B program at a level until they are proficient at those workouts and then move on to the similarly structured program at the next level. In terms of making the greatest improvements in the pool, the second or third plan would be best.

A definitive description of the type of swimmer who would benefit most from each program is virtually impossible. The range of experience, goals, situations, and abilities all play into which program is best suited for a swimmer at any given time. However, the introduction of each program provides a few notes explaining which type of swimmer was in mind when the program was designed.

The workouts are abbreviated in the program charts as follows:

Fit     Building Swim Fitness workouts from chapter 5

Base     Building a Base workouts from chapter 6

AT     Increasing Anaerobic Threshold workouts from chapter 7

Spd     Increasing Speed workouts from chapter 8

IM     Swimming the IM workouts from chapter 9

# Level 1A

The first program in level 1 is the easiest of the dozen in this book and is designed for beginning swimmers. After building up their swim fitness as described in chapter 3, newcomers will be challenged by the variety and distance but should feel comfortable incorporating interval training and the use of pace clocks into their workouts.

This four-week program is well suited for swimmers with little to no experience for two reasons. One, the program is based on the first two workouts in each chapter of part II. The workouts range in length from 600 yards to 3,000 yards, though all but one are 2,500 yards or less. Two, this program involves swimming just three times a week. Taking one or two days off between sessions should give the body enough time to recuperate before hitting the pool again. By swimming consistently and continuing to challenge yourself, you'll notice gains in comfort and improvement after only a few weeks.

The most challenging aspect of this program for newer swimmers likely will be the two 2,500-yard IM workouts. If your technique or endurance for one or more of the backstroke, breaststroke, and butterfly is not well developed, it might be necessary to alter or replace these workouts. The best course of action is to follow the workouts as closely as possible, substituting the freestyle for the difficult strokes so that you continue working on the IM even if you're not comfortable with one or two of the four strokes. The other option is to replace the IM workouts with base 1 or base 2.

| | Sun | Mon | Tue | Wed | Thu | Fri | Sat |
|---|---|---|---|---|---|---|---|
| **Week 1** | | Base 2 2,500 yd Page 120 | | Fit 1 600 yd Page 105 | | Spd 1 1,500 yd Page 149 | |
| **Week 2** | | Base 1 2,500 yd Page 119 | | AT 2 2,500 yd Page 134 | | Fit 2 600 yd Page 106 | |
| **Week 3** | | IM 1 2,500 yd Page 165 | | Fit 3 600 yd Page 107 | | Spd 2 1,500 yd Page 150 | |
| **Week 4** | | Base 3 3,000 yd Page 121 | | AT 1 2,500 yd Page 133 | | IM 2 2,500 yd Page 166 | |

# Level 1B

Level 1B differs from level 1A in two primary ways. First, this four-week program calls for swimming four times a week instead of three. Second, to keep swimmers progressing gradually, the average total distance of each workout is slightly higher than at level 1A. Again, most sessions are 2,500 yards or less, but a few are at 3,000 yards.

Level 1B is best suited for two types of swimmers. Newer swimmers who built up their swim fitness following the guidelines in chapter 3 and followed level 1A at least twice should be prepared for the longer and more frequent workouts. Also, swimmers who are getting back in the pool after several months or years off would do well to begin with this program. Both groups will enjoy obvious improvement after a dozen or so consistent and challenging workouts.

Swimming four days a week means you will swim back-to-back days at least once. Notice that in all but one of those instances in this program, a fitness workout is the second of the successive sessions. Because they are shorter in length and lack the intensity of the AT, speed, or IM workouts, swimming on consecutive days should be manageable. Both IM sessions are 2,500 yards. If you can swim two or three of the strokes well enough, push yourself to follow as much of the workout as possible while replacing part or all of the yardage that calls for the more difficult stroke(s) with one(s) in which you are more proficient. Replace them with the 3,000-yard base 3 or base 4 if necessary.

|        | Sun | Mon | Tue | Wed | Thu | Fri | Sat |
|--------|-----|-----|-----|-----|-----|-----|-----|
| **Week 1** | Base 1<br>2,500 yd<br>Page 119 | Fit 2<br>600 yd<br>Page 106 | | Spd 1<br>1,500 yd<br>Page 149 | | AT 2<br>2,500 yd<br>Page 134 | |
| **Week 2** | Base 2<br>2,500 yd<br>Page 120 | Fit 1<br>600 yd<br>Page 105 | | IM 1<br>2,500 yd<br>Page 165 | | AT 1<br>2,500 yd<br>Page 133 | |
| **Week 3** | Base 3<br>3,000 yd<br>Page 121 | Spd 2<br>1,500 yd<br>Page 150 | | IM 2<br>2,500 yd<br>Page 166 | | Fit 3<br>600 yd<br>Page 107 | |
| **Week 4** | AT 3<br>3,000 yd<br>Page 135 | Fit 4<br>1,000 yd<br>Page 108 | | Spd 3<br>1,500 yd<br>Page 151 | | Base 4<br>3,000 yd<br>Page 122 | |

# Level 2A

Level 2A is another four-week program for swimmers who can get to the pool three times a week. This level is the natural progression for swimmers who have either completed level 1A a few times and are ready to continue their steady gains in improvement or for those who have completed level 1B two or more times but are unable to swim four times a week in the immediate future. This program also works well for more accomplished fitness swimmers with limited time to dedicate to their workouts, or for those who enjoy incorporating other fitness activities into their schedules. Experienced swimmers who are pressed for time, or competitors who need a break from their normally intense workouts, will enjoy the change of pace and distance of level 2A.

Half of the workouts are either 3,000 yards or 3,500 yards, but the lack of intensity of the longer base workouts should make the increased distance an appropriate progression. Again, if the IM workouts are a struggle, substitute yardage of the more difficult strokes with an easier stroke, or replace the workouts with base 3 or base 4.

| | Sun | Mon | Tue | Wed | Thu | Fri | Sat |
|---|---|---|---|---|---|---|---|
| **Week 1** | | Base 4 3,000 yd Page 122 | | Fit 3 600 yd Page 107 | | IM 2 2,500 yd Page 166 | |
| **Week 2** | | Base 3 3,000 yd Page 121 | | AT 3 3,000 yd Page 135 | | Fit 4 1,000 yd Page 108 | |
| **Week 3** | | Spd 4 2,000 yd Page 152 | | Base 5 3,500 yd Page 123 | | AT 4 3,000 yd Page 136 | |
| **Week 4** | | IM 3 3,000 yd Page 167 | | Fit 5 1,000 yd Page 109 | | Spd 5 2,000 yd Page 153 | |

# Level 2B

Completing any of the previous programs—especially level 1B or 2A—or their equivalents one or more times prepares you for level 2B. Once swimmers can finish this program exactly as it's written, they can begin to feel confident that they aren't beginners any more, even if they still feel new to the sport. Experienced swimmers also might find that the length, frequency, or intensity of workouts in this program fit well into their schedules or training plans.

Swimming the 2,500-yard IM workout in the first week will give you the confidence to move up to the 3,000-yarders in the second and fourth weeks. Alter strokes if necessary, or replace the workouts with base 5, base 6, AT 3, or AT 4. The wide variety of workouts in this program will keep you progressing in fitness, comfort in the sport, confidence, and performance.

|  | Sun | Mon | Tue | Wed | Thu | Fri | Sat |
|---|---|---|---|---|---|---|---|
| **Week 1** | Base 3 3,000 yd Page 121 | Fit 4 1,000 yd Page 108 |  | IM 2 2,500 yd Page 166 |  | Spd 3 1,500 yd Page 151 |  |
| **Week 2** | Base 4 3,000 yd Page 122 | AT 3 3,000 yd Page 135 |  | Fit 3 600 yd Page 107 |  | IM 3 3,000 yd Page 167 |  |
| **Week 3** | Spd 4 2,000 yd Page 152 | Base 6 3,500 yd Page 124 |  | AT 4 3,000 yd Page 136 |  | Fit 5 1,000 yd Page 109 |  |
| **Week 4** | IM 4 3,000 yd Page 168 | Base 5 3,500 yd Page 123 |  | Fit 6 1,000 yd Page 110 |  | AT 5 3,500 yd Page 137 |  |

# Level 3A

This three-times-a-week program is no lightweight. It is the first six-week program and the first to introduce a 4,000-yard workout—base 7 in the final week. Because of the increased distances and intensity of these workouts compared to those at level 1 and level 2, the body will need the additional time to adapt to the higher workload before it's ready to move on to the next level.

A few rounds through level 2A or 2B should prepare virtually any swimmer for this program. That progression should result in fairly solid development of all aspects of swim fitness, including base, anaerobic threshold, speed, and individual medley. Workouts at these distances will take most experienced swimmers about an hour to complete, so level 3 programs will probably be among the most popular. Most masters swimmers will fall into this category, as will swimmers who have months or years of swimming fitness packed into their muscles.

As usual, the toughest workouts—a 4,000-yard base and two 3,500-yard IMs—come toward the end of the program. Most swimmers should be able to follow the IM workouts to a T if they've pushed themselves in previous programs, so alter them, if necessary, instead of replacing them. Accomplished swimmers should continue to challenge themselves to lower their base as they work through this program.

| | Sun | Mon | Tue | Wed | Thu | Fri | Sat |
|---|---|---|---|---|---|---|---|
| **Week 1** | | Base 4<br>3,000 yd<br>Page 122 | | Fit 4<br>1,000 yd<br>Page 108 | | IM 3<br>3,000 yd<br>Page 167 | |
| **Week 2** | | Base 5<br>3,500 yd<br>Page 123 | | AT 4<br>3,000 yd<br>Page 136 | | Spd 4<br>2,000 yd<br>Page 152 | |
| **Week 3** | | AT 5<br>3,500 yd<br>Page 137 | | IM 4<br>3,000 yd<br>Page 168 | | Fit 5<br>1,000 yd<br>Page 109 | |
| **Week 4** | | Base 6<br>3,500 yd<br>Page 124 | | Spd 6<br>2,000 yd<br>Page 154 | | AT 6<br>3,500 yd<br>Page 138 | |
| **Week 5** | | IM 5<br>3,500 yd<br>Page 169 | | Fit 6<br>1,000 yd<br>Page 110 | | Spd 5<br>2,000 yd<br>Page 153 | |
| **Week 6** | | Base 7<br>4,000 yd<br>Page 125 | | Fit 7<br>1,500 yd<br>Page 111 | | IM 6<br>3,500 yd<br>Page 170 | |

# Level 3B

The level 3B program is reliably versatile for a wide range of swimmers, with a solid four-times-a-week rotation based on an also solid 3,500-yard distance built into a six-week plan. The distance and frequency of these workouts will challenge swimmers moving up from level 2, enable good swimmers to maintain their level of fitness, and provide a slight break for those who normally swim more than 4,000 yards per workout.

Once swimmers are progressing through the levels, they won't be surprised that workouts at the base length are only the foundation and not the majority of the program. The average total distance of the workouts is such that most swimmers will need about an hour to complete them, with a goal of continuing to refine their strokes and lower their bases. Swimmers starting at level 1 and advancing through level 2 might need more time before they're able to swim faster and spend less time at the wall. The level 3B program could also be perfect for long-distance swimmers who find themselves cramped for time or wanting to take things easier for a few weeks.

Level 3

|  | Sun | Mon | Tue | Wed | Thu | Fri | Sat |
|---|---|---|---|---|---|---|---|
| **Week 1** | Base 4<br>3,000 yd<br>Page 122 | Fit 4<br>1,000 yd<br>Page 108 |  | IM 3<br>3,000 yd<br>Page 167 |  | AT 4<br>3,000 yd<br>Page 136 |  |
| **Week 2** | Base 5<br>3,500 yd<br>Page 123 | Spd 4<br>2,000 yd<br>Page 152 |  | Fit 5<br>1,000 yd<br>Page 109 |  | IM 4<br>3,000 yd<br>Page 168 |  |
| **Week 3** | AT 5<br>3,500 yd<br>Page 137 | Fit 6<br>1,000 yd<br>Page 110 |  | Base 6<br>3,500 yd<br>Page 124 |  | Spd 5<br>2,000 yd<br>Page 153 |  |
| **Week 4** | IM 5<br>3,500 yd<br>Page 169 | AT 6<br>3,500 yd<br>Page 138 |  | Base 8<br>4,000 yd<br>Page 126 |  | Fit 7<br>1,500 yd<br>Page 111 |  |
| **Week 5** | Spd 6<br>2,000 yd<br>Page 154 | IM 6<br>3,500 yd<br>Page 170 |  | Fit 8<br>1,500 yd<br>Page 112 |  | AT 8<br>4,000 yd<br>Page 140 |  |
| **Week 6** | Base 7<br>4,000 yd<br>Page 125 | Spd 7<br>2,500 yd<br>Page 155 |  | IM 7<br>4,000 yd<br>Page 171 |  | AT 7<br>4,000 yd<br>Page 139 |  |

# Level 4A

Swimmers who choose to follow level 4A can consider themselves nothing less than proficient. The jump to 4,000- and 4,500-yard workouts puts most of the workouts into the relatively serious category for nonelite athletes, which can take up to one-and-a-half hours to complete. Understandably, the satisfaction that comes from completing a level 4 program is typically quite high.

The range in workout distances is more varied in 4A than in previous programs both in number of distances represented as well as the difference between the shortest and longest workouts. This variety should help keep swimmers engaged mentally and improving physically in all aspects of swim fitness. The relative abundance of fitness and base workouts (9), combined with the relatively few IM workouts (3), keep the program manageable for those progressing through the levels. The order of the workouts in each week should keep the muscles fresh throughout the program.

| | Sun | Mon | Tue | Wed | Thu | Fri | Sat |
|---|---|---|---|---|---|---|---|
| **Week 1** | | Base 6 3,500 yd Page 124 | | Fit 7 1,500 yd Page 111 | | AT 6 3,500 yd Page 138 | |
| **Week 2** | | IM 4 3,000 yd Page 168 | | Spd 6 2,000 yd Page 154 | | Base 8 4,000 yd Page 126 | |
| **Week 3** | | AT 7 4,000 yd Page 139 | | Base 7 4,000 yd Page 125 | | Fit 6 1,000 yd Page 110 | |
| **Week 4** | | IM 5 3,500 yd Page 169 | | Spd 7 2,500 yd Page 155 | | AT 8 4,000 yd Page 140 | |
| **Week 5** | | Base 6 3,500 yd Page 124 | | Fit 9 1,500 yd Page 113 | | IM 6 3,500 yd Page 170 | |
| **Week 6** | | AT 9 4,500 yd Page 141 | | Base 9 4,500 yd Page 127 | | Fit 8 1,500 yd Page 112 | |

# Level 4B

The last of the moderate yet challenging programs is level 4B, which arranges relatively long workouts into a four-times-a-week routine for capable swimmers. On average, the workouts take 75 to 90 minutes to complete, so the commitment level is sizeable—as is a swimmer's levels of satisfaction and confidence after completing this program.

Like level 4A, 4B calls for a wide range of workouts. There are more base sessions in this program than any other type and in any previous program. The five easier fitness workouts are countered by five difficult IM sessions, and four each of AT and speed workouts lend not only variety but intensity to get the heart rate racing as swimmers build and use easy speed. Pay attention to effort level in this program so you can bounce back appropriately after workouts, especially those that fall on consecutive days.

| | Sun | Mon | Tue | Wed | Thu | Fri | Sat |
|---|---|---|---|---|---|---|---|
| **Week 1** | Base 6 3,500 yd Page 124 | Fit 6 1,000 yd Page 110 | | IM 4 3,000 yd Page 168 | | AT 6 3,500 yd Page 138 | |
| **Week 2** | Spd 6 2,000 yd Page 154 | Fit 8 1,500 yd Page 112 | | Base 7 4,000 yd Page 125 | | IM 5 3,500 yd Page 169 | |
| **Week 3** | AT 8 4,000 yd Page 140 | Base 8 4,000 yd Page 126 | | Spd 7 2,500 yd Page 155 | | Fit 7 1,500 yd Page 111 | |
| **Week 4** | IM 6 3,500 yd Page 170 | AT 7 4,000 yd Page 139 | | Base 9 4,500 yd Page 127 | | Spd 8 2,500 yd Page 156 | |
| **Week 5** | Base 10 4,500 yd Page 128 | Fit 9 1,500 yd Page 113 | | IM 7 4,000 yd Page 171 | | AT 9 4,500 yd Page 141 | |
| **Week 6** | Base 8 4,000 yd Page 126 | Spd 9 2,500 yd Page 157 | | Fit 10 2,000 yd Page 114 | | IM 8 4,000 yd Page 172 | |

# Level 5A

The first of four programs designed for the serious, accomplished swimmer, level 5A makes the jump in base workout distance (4,500 yards) and program length (eight weeks), but that's not all. This is the first level in which the shorter of the two programs calls for swimming four days a week instead of three. The combination makes for a difficult two-month regimen.

Many swimmers progressing through the levels might find it necessary to follow the programs at level 4 several times to be fully ready to tackle level 5A. Hardcore swimmers will enjoy the high number of AT, speed, and IM workouts that makes the program challenging. Anticipation of improved performance should keep motivation high as well. Be sure to keep effort levels within the appropriate range to avoid burnout, overextended muscles, and injury.

Level 5

|  | Sun | Mon | Tue | Wed | Thu | Fri | Sat |
|---|---|---|---|---|---|---|---|
| **Week 1** | Base 8<br>4,000 yd<br>Page 126 | Fit 7<br>1,500 yd<br>Page 111 |  | IM 5<br>3,500 yd<br>Page 169 |  | AT 8<br>4,000 yd<br>Page 140 |  |
| **Week 2** | Base 7<br>4,000 yd<br>Page 125 | Spd 8<br>2,500 yd<br>Page 156 |  | AT 7<br>4,000 yd<br>Page 139 |  | Fit 8<br>1,500 yd<br>Page 112 |  |
| **Week 3** | IM 6<br>3,500 yd<br>Page 170 | Fit 10<br>2,000 yd<br>Page 114 |  | Base 9<br>4,500 yd<br>Page 127 |  | Spd 7<br>2,500 yd<br>Page 155 |  |
| **Week 4** | IM 8<br>4,000 yd<br>Page 172 | Fit 9<br>1,500 yd<br>Page 113 |  | AT 10<br>4,500 yd<br>Page 143 |  | Base 8<br>4,000 yd<br>Page 126 |  |
| **Week 5** | Spd 9<br>2,500 yd<br>Page 157 | IM 7<br>4,000 yd<br>Page 171 |  | Fit 10<br>2,000 yd<br>Page 114 |  | AT 9<br>4,500 yd<br>Page 141 |  |
| **Week 6** | Base 10<br>4,500 yd<br>Page 128 | Fit 11<br>2,000 yd<br>Page 115 |  | Spd 10<br>3,000 yd<br>Page 158 |  | AT 10<br>4,500 yd<br>Page 143 |  |
| **Week 7** | Base 9<br>4,500 yd<br>Page 127 | AT 11<br>5,000 yd<br>Page 144 |  | Spd 11<br>3,000 yd<br>Page 160 |  | IM 9<br>4,500 yd<br>Page 173 |  |
| **Week 8** | Base 11<br>5,000 yd<br>Page 129 | Fit 11<br>2,000 yd<br>Page 115 |  | IM 10<br>4,500 yd<br>Page 175 |  | Spd 12<br>3,000 yd<br>Page 161 |  |

# Level 5B

The hard-easy principle as applied to workouts on back-to-back days comes into play at level 5B, the first of two programs that have swimmers in the pool five times a week. With only two days off, you can't help but swim on consecutive days at least three times. This is tough but very possible with the steady, progressive development and confidence that rising through levels 1 through 4 or years of consistent swimming yields. Following level 4B should be a prerequisite for almost any swimmer wanting to tackle level 5B.

Accomplished swimmers who can undertake level 5B will enjoy the challenge that longer AT, speed, and IM workouts provide. The variation of speed, effort, and stroke breaks up the long base workouts, and the shorter fitness workouts provide a much needed physical and mental break each week of the program. The result is a highly fit and competitive swimmer. Athletes at this level might tend to push themselves too hard, which often has an adverse effect on improvement. Swimming the workouts as they are written—especially the effort levels—is increasingly important at this level.

|  | Sun | Mon | Tue | Wed | Thu | Fri | Sat |
|---|---|---|---|---|---|---|---|
| **Week 1** | Base 7 4,000 yd Page 125 | Fit 8 1,500 yd Page 112 |  | Spd 7 2,500 yd Page 155 | AT 7 4,000 yd Page 139 |  | IM 5 3,500 yd Page 169 |
| **Week 2** | Base 8 4,000 yd Page 126 | Spd 9 2,500 yd Page 157 |  | Fit 7 1,500 yd Page 111 | AT 8 4,000 yd Page 140 |  | Base 9 4,500 yd Page 127 |
| **Week 3** | IM 6 3,500 yd Page 170 | Fit 9 1,500 yd Page 113 |  | Base 7 4,000 yd Page 125 | Spd 8 2,500 yd Page 156 |  | AT 9 4,500 yd Page 141 |
| **Week 4** | Fit 10 2,000 yd Page 114 | IM 8 4,000 yd Page 172 |  | Base 10 4,500 yd Page 128 | AT 10 4,500 yd Page 143 |  | Spd 10 3,000 yd Page 158 |
| **Week 5** | IM 7 4,000 yd Page 171 | Base 9 4,500 yd Page 127 |  | AT 11 5,000 yd Page 144 | Fit 11 2,000 yd Page 115 |  | Spd 9 2,500 yd Page 157 |
| **Week 6** | Base 8 4,000 yd Page 126 | Fit 10 2,000 yd Page 114 |  | IM 9 4,500 yd Page 173 | AT 9 4,500 yd Page 141 |  | Spd 11 3,000 yd Page 160 |
| **Week 7** | Fit 12 2,000 yd Page 116 | Base 10 4,500 yd Page 128 |  | Spd 12 3,000 yd Page 161 | IM 10 4,500 yd Page 175 |  | AT 10 4,500 yd Page 143 |
| **Week 8** | Base 11 5,000 yd Page 129 | Spd 11 3,000 yd Page 160 |  | IM 11 5,000 yd Page 176 | Fit 11 2,000 yd Page 115 |  | AT 11 5,000 yd Page 144 |

Level 5

# Level 6A

If you have been disciplined enough to advance to the level 6 programs, or can already swim at this level, give yourself a pat on the back and take time to relish the accomplishment. You've done something few swimmers can do. Swimming 4,500- to 5,000-yard workouts multiple times a week, including IMs and shorter but high-intensity speed sessions, is tough to achieve. Following the workouts as they are written, especially staying within the maximum heart rate zones, is key to optimal development and to an injury-free program.

An increasingly limited number of workouts in part II are long enough to challenge swimmers at this level, but only five are repeated in level 6A. The variety keeps workouts fresh in several ways. The distance of the workouts ranges from 1,200-yard fitness sessions to 5,000-yarders in the base, AT, and IM chapters. Twenty-seven different workouts are represented. No week contains two workouts from the same chapter.

Level 6A swimmers tend to be significantly motivated, whether because of pride in their fitness level or in their goals of competition. Most athletes at this level are competing at an elite masters level.

|  | Sun | Mon | Tue | Wed | Thu | Fri | Sat |
|---|---|---|---|---|---|---|---|
| **Week 1** | Base 8 4,000 yd Page 126 | Fit 9 1,500 yd Page 113 |  | IM 6 3,500 yd Page 170 |  | AT 8 4,000 yd Page 140 |  |
| **Week 2** | Base 9 4,500 yd Page 127 | Spd 7 2,500 yd Page 155 |  | AT 7 4,000 yd Page 139 |  | IM 7 4,000 yd Page 171 |  |
| **Week 3** | Base 10 4,500 yd Page 128 | Fit 10 2,000 yd Page 114 |  | Spd 8 2,500 yd Page 156 |  | AT 9 4,500 yd Page 141 |  |
| **Week 4** | IM 8 4,000 yd Page 172 | Spd 9 2,500 yd Page 157 |  | AT 10 4,500 yd Page 143 |  | Base 11 5,000 yd Page 129 |  |
| **Week 5** | IM 9 4,500 yd Page 173 | Fit 11 2,000 yd Page 115 |  | Base 12 5,000 yd Page 130 |  | AT 11 5,000 yd Page 144 |  |
| **Week 6** | Base 11 5,000 yd Page 129 | Spd 11 3,000 yd Page 160 |  | AT 12 5,000 yd Page 145 |  | Fit 10 2,000 yd Page 114 |  |
| **Week 7** | IM 10 4,500 yd Page 175 | Fit 12 2,000 yd Page 116 |  | Base 10 4,500 yd Page 128 |  | Spd 10 3,000 yd Page 158 |  |
| **Week 8** | IM 11 5,000 yd Page 176 | AT 11 5,000 yd Page 144 |  | Base 12 5,000 yd Page 130 |  | Fit 11 2,000 yd Page 115 |  |

# Level 6B

Congratulations. Once you have reached level 6B, you are in the upper echelon of the swimming world, topped perhaps only by swimmers competing for their countries in international meets. There's a good chance some of you are knocking on that door yourselves, or were at some point in your swimming careers. Precision in training, nutrition, time management, and commitment have brought you to this level of accomplishment, which is what it takes to swim 4,500 to 5,000 yards several times a week.

Level 6B is a collection of workouts pulled equally from the five chapters in part II. More than half of the workouts are 4,000 yards or more (23 in all), and even the majority of the speed sessions are 3,000 yards. Eight fitness workouts are strategically placed to give your body a break from the high effort required by the program. Thirteen workouts appear more than once to keep the program as challenging as possible.

|  | Sun | Mon | Tue | Wed | Thu | Fri | Sat |
|---|---|---|---|---|---|---|---|
| **Week 1** | Base 9 4,500 yd Page 127 | Fit 8 1,500 yd Page 112 |  | Spd 8 2,500 yd Page 156 | IM 6 3,500 yd Page 170 |  | AT 8 4,000 yd Page 140 |
| **Week 2** | Base 8 4,000 yd Page 126 | Spd 10 3,000 yd Page 158 |  | AT 10 4,500 yd Page 143 | IM 8 4,000 yd Page 172 |  | Fit 9 1,500 yd Page 113 |
| **Week 3** | AT 9 4,500 yd Page 141 | Base 10 4,500 yd Page 128 |  | IM 7 4,000 yd Page 171 | Fit 10 2,000 yd Page 114 |  | Spd 9 2,500 yd Page 157 |
| **Week 4** | Base 11 5,000 yd Page 129 | IM 9 4,500 yd Page 173 |  | AT 11 5,000 yd Page 144 | Spd 10 3,000 yd Page 158 |  | Fit 11 2,000 yd Page 115 |
| **Week 5** | Base 12 5,000 yd Page 130 | AT 12 5,000 yd Page 145 |  | Fit 12 2,000 yd Page 116 | Spd 9 2,500 yd Page 157 |  | IM 9 4,500 yd Page 173 |
| **Week 6** | Base 9 4,500 yd Page 127 | Fit 10 2,000 yd Page 114 |  | IM 10 4,500 yd Page 175 | AT 10 4,500 yd Page 143 |  | Spd 11 3,000 yd Page 160 |
| **Week 7** | IM 11 5,000 yd Page 176 | Fit 11 2,000 yd Page 115 |  | Base 10 4,500 yd Page 128 | Spd 12 3,000 yd Page 161 |  | AT 11 5,000 yd Page 144 |
| **Week 8** | Base 12 5,000 yd Page 130 | Fit 12 2,000 yd Page 116 |  | AT 12 5,000 yd Page 145 | Spd 11 3,000 yd Page 160 |  | IM 12 5,000 yd Page 177 |

# chapter 11

# Training for a Race

The instruction, workouts, and programs in this book provide guidance to improve swim fitness, overall fitness, stroke technique, muscle tone and endurance, and flexibility. Swimming longer and harder workouts begins to take less effort than shorter and easier workouts required just weeks or months before. Your body feels taut, your mind clear, and your spirits high. As great as those benefits are, though, they might not be enough. The aspirations of some swimmers are even higher: to focus, train, and prepare as well as possible to compete in a specific meet or race. Swimming consistently and moving up through the program levels will help considerably with that goal. But to arrive at a particular meet or race ready to take advantage of the weeks and months of training, a specific plan tailored to your objectives, abilities, and particular race or races is required.

Training for a race is quite individualized. In all my years of swimming, no two people had exactly the same training program. Workouts would often be the same, and some swimmers' programs might be similar to those of others, but there are so many factors to consider in a well-designed training plan that it's virtually impossible, or at least highly unlikely, for one swimmer's program to perfectly suit another swimmer. For starters, each race or event calls for a specific plan. Sprinters require a different type of fitness and training than middle-distance swimmers, who have different needs from distance swimmers. Even within those categories are minor distinctions. For example, if a 100 freestyler trained with the 50 freestylers, he very well may be the fastest in the first half of the race but will probably fade considerably over the second 50. Swimmers themselves are different as well, even those who swim exactly the same events. One 200 IMer might have natural speed in all four strokes but struggle with endurance. Her teammate might have excellent stamina but lack efficiency in the butterfly.

One breaststroke specialist might need more work on upper-body mechanics, another on the kick.

Given just those few examples, it's easy to see how including race-training programs for a broad audience is impossible, or at the very least ineffective. But that doesn't mean you racers are out of luck and must continue to guess at the distances, speeds, and types of workouts to swim in the months preceding a big event. The guidelines in chapter 3, such as building swim fitness, interval training, and gauging effort, and the four principles on which the programs in chapter 10 are based are important pieces to the training puzzle. By combining them with the information in this chapter on the four phases of a training program and the importance of rest, any swimmer can design a plan with the best chance of setting a personal record or making the finals in an upcoming race.

# Training Phases

Because of the body's ability to adapt to the demands placed on it and the range of energy systems used during a performance, the long-term preparation for a meet or race should be planned carefully based on the training principle of periodization. Periodization breaks a training season—defined as the time between the beginning of structured training and the last or most important race on your schedule—into distinct phases that capitalize on the benefits of the body's adaptive response to workouts and target different aspects of fitness. Each period or phase of training varies in focus to lead the body on a gradual but continual climb toward peak fitness. Intensity builds in successive phases, so following the phases in order is critical for the best and safest results. Otherwise, the body might not be properly conditioned to endure the rigors of the later phases. It might be necessary to prioritize your races and train through the lesser ones to maximize improvement for the most important ones.

The four primary training phases in swimming, once swim fitness is achieved, are building a base, improving anaerobic threshold, increasing speed, and tapering. The ideal amount of time that swimmers should spend within each training phase is amazingly consistent regardless of ability or experience. Although more seasoned swimmers might not need quite as much time to build their base as newer swimmers, the veterans operate under the same physiological principles that dictate the body's reaction to training. Veterans and newcomers alike will benefit from periodizing their training programs.

The first phase, building a base, should comprise approximately 36 percent of the total time of training before the featured event. Time spent improving both anaerobic threshold and speed should be about 27 percent each, and the tapering phase should be 10 percent or two weeks, whichever is shorter. Table 11.1 provides sample breakdowns of training phases based on

**Table 11.1  Periodization of Training Phases**

| Training phase | Training programs by length | | | | |
| --- | --- | --- | --- | --- | --- |
| | 17 weeks (4 months) | 22 weeks (5 months) | 26 weeks (6 months) | 30 weeks (7 months) | 34 weeks (8 months) |
| **Building a base** | 6 weeks (35%) | 8 weeks (36%) | 10 weeks (38%) | 11 weeks (37%) | 12 weeks (35%) |
| **Improving anaerobic threshold** | 5 weeks (29%) | 6 weeks (27%) | 7 weeks (27%) | 9 weeks (30%) | 10 weeks (29%) |
| **Increasing speed** | 5 weeks (29%) | 6 weeks (27%) | 7 weeks (27%) | 8 weeks (27%) | 10 weeks (29%) |
| **Tapering** | 1 week (6%) | 2 weeks (10%) | 2 weeks (8%) | 2 weeks (7%) | 2 weeks (6%) |

common training seasons. If the date for a race or meet is within 17 weeks (four months), it's best to have a good base already. Otherwise, you run the risk of injury because the increase in intensity and speed comes more quickly than the body's ability to fully adapt to it.

The breakdown of workouts swum will vary somewhat during the weeks of each training phase. The latter stages of each phase should be used to transition gradually into the next phase. The majority of workouts during each phase are specific to that phase, but other types of workouts are mixed in to maintain or build your fitness in those areas. For example, Building a Base workouts will be swum in every phase to maintain the endurance you have established, but the number of those workouts will continue to decrease as you move from phase to phase. The length of workouts you should be swimming is also important. Each chapter in part II included workouts of six different lengths. In general, stick with similarly numbered workouts among the chapters. For instance, all Workout 3s are comparable in difficulty based on the fitness focus although they might not be comparable in distance swum. For instance, Building a Base 3 is 3,000 yards, whereas Increasing Speed 3 is 1,500 yards. But the higher intensity level of the latter compensates for the lesser distance and makes the degree of difficulty similar. The following sections describe each training phase in detail.

# Building a Base

As discussed in chapter 6, building a base of cardiovascular and muscular endurance will increase your ability to swim at a steady rate for extended distances and periods of time. It's the most important phase of the season, as indicated by the larger percentage of time spent in the phase. Establishing solid endurance through swimming longer distances at a moderate pace, the hallmark of Building a Base workouts, gives you the strong foundation on which the other phases can be developed. It will also help prevent injuries by preparing the body's muscles, ligaments, and tendons for the exertion of the faster tempos and increased intensity that follow. A good foundation of swim fitness is a prerequisite to this phase.

The first 50 percent of this phase should include only Building a Base workouts from chapter 6 on a base that keeps the heart rate between 70 and 85 percent of its maximum. Halfway through the phase, after the body has adapted to the workouts and the base has been established, begin to incorporate individual medley workouts from chapter 9. The IM sessions will provide some variety to the training regimen and also help strengthen your base by taxing the muscles in slightly different ways. They should displace about 25 percent of the base workouts during the third quarter of this phase and should be chosen based on physical and technical ability. Almost all swimmers will favor certain strokes over others, so begin with the ones that feature your better strokes. As you gain proficiency and endurance, progress to workouts that include longer distances and more difficult strokes. Be aware of two points when beginning to swim IM workouts. First, IM workouts are tough, so don't expect to master them in a few short months. Second, the purpose of this phase is to build endurance. The IM workouts should help with that goal, so keep the heart rate between 70 and 85 percent of MHR.

The final 25 percent of the phase will maintain its focus on endurance. About 70 percent of the workouts will be base and 20 percent IM. The remaining 10 percent are anaerobic threshold workouts to help the body's transition from the even-paced endurance work to the faster tempo and varied rates in the next phase. Anaerobic threshold workouts can vary in difficulty depending on the ratio of lower ES distance to higher ES distance. This phase should consist of the easier anaerobic threshold workouts that feature the most distance swum at lower effort.

The base phase is just as important for sprinters as it is for distance swimmers. Although during all other phases a sprinter's total distance swum will be approximately 60 percent of a distance swimmer's, early in a season everyone will swim virtually the same distances. Developing that base of aerobic and muscular endurance will carry any swimmer safely and successfully through the season.

## Increasing Anaerobic Threshold

After building a solid base of endurance, the next step in training for a race is developing the body's ability to swim at a faster pace for a longer period of time—easy speed, as described in chapter 7. Increasing the amount of time you can swim fast is critical to success in competition. Physiologically, there is a speed at which the effort changes from aerobic (the muscles' need for oxygen can be met indefinitely) to anaerobic (the body cannot carry adequate quantities of oxygen to the muscles, and the swimmer can sustain a given pace for only a minute or so). That speed varies by individual and is based on the body's ability to deliver oxygen efficiently. The purpose of this phase is to increase the efficiency with which the body supplies oxygen to the muscles. Doing so increases the speed, effort levels, and duration the body can continue supplying sufficient amounts of oxygen to the muscles.

The bulk of workouts in this phase should be spent swimming anaerobic threshold workouts from chapter 7 that build your capacity for easy speed. The mix within these workouts of total distance at a higher intensity (up to about 90 percent of MHR) and a more moderate intensity (about 70 percent of MHR) trains the heart to pump more blood containing more oxygen through the blood vessels at a faster rate to keep up with demand. Start with workouts that have the greatest percentage of lower ES distance and gradually shift that percentage each week so that by the end of the phase you're swimming workouts with more distance at the higher ES.

For the first half of the phase, 25 percent of the workouts should be base from chapter 6 and 15 percent should be IM from chapter 9. (The remaining 60 percent should be the anaerobic threshold workouts just described.) If you followed the previous phase properly, you will have developed a strong endurance base. Maintaining that base is not as difficult as building it, but it still requires some attention so that those gains are not lost.

During the second half of the phase, the emphasis shifts to the tempo requirements of the speed phase. The percentages of base and IM workouts decrease to 20 percent and 10 percent, respectively, and 10 percent of the workout should be spent on speed work. The endurance workouts should decrease in distance and intensity as the intensity of anaerobic threshold and sprint workouts increases—this carves out a bit of room in your energy stores that you'll need to ramp up the effort level required by those workouts. Start with speed workouts that are one step shorter in distance compared to the base and IM workouts.

# Increasing Speed

Once you hit the phase in which speed is the emphasis, you're about two-thirds of the way through training for the race or meet! The goal in this phase is to maintain the great base of endurance you've worked so hard to build while increasing your stroke tempo so that you're ready to swim at maximum speed in the race. Walking (or swimming, if you will) that fine line of maintaining endurance and building speed can be done with the proper combination of workouts.

This is the only phase in which the breakdown of workouts remains consistent over the entire phase. Speed workouts from chapter 8 comprise 50 percent of the sessions. After having eased into speed work during the end of the anaerobic threshold phase, make the step up in distance if you're comfortable and competent with the higher intensity and speeds. This should mean the level of difficulty of the various types of workouts—indicated by similar workout numbers—is again in synch. Anaerobic threshold and base workouts each make up 20 percent of the sessions, with the remaining 10 percent coming from the IM chapter. That breakdown clearly puts the focus on tempo without neglecting the need to maintain that base of endurance and keeps the point at which effort becomes anaerobic as high as possible. The endurance workouts should be of moderate distance—perhaps 500 to 1,000 yards (about 450-900 meters) shorter than your longest workout in the base phase—and remain in the ES 6 range. Both factors will keep them difficult enough to keep the aerobic base from slipping but not so difficult as to really break down the muscles.

Although you'll be swimming at maximum or near maximum effort in the speed workouts, the rest between each sprint allows full recovery within the workout and, to a lesser degree, between workouts. The amount of rest you'll be getting in the majority of these workouts sets the stage for the tapering phase.

## Tapering

Swimmers love the days immediately before a big race. These days include progressively shorter workouts, faster tempos, and lots of rest. By slowly cutting back on training intensity and distance while maintaining the endurance, anaerobic threshold, speed, and feel for the water you've worked so hard to gain, the body can recuperate fully from the weeks of grueling workouts without losing any fitness. If all goes according to plan, swimmers arrive at the race very fit, very rested, and very fast.

Throughout your training you have been pushing and pushing your body to get stronger every day, to become as fit and fast as possible. The rest in between each workout should have been enough to allow the next workout to be performed as designed, but not enough to allow complete recovery. After all, if the body has completely recovered, there's no longer a need for it to continue adapting! But the body cannot continue to build in training intensity forever. Eventually, fitness will peak, plateau, and then decline. The goal of tapering is to plan for that peak to arrive on the day of the big race. This phase is all about fine-tuning the body's fitness level and the stroke at race pace.

Taper workouts should be similar in breakdown to the workouts in the sprint phase. The decrease in distance comes almost exclusively from the main set, and distance in the sprint set should actually increase by 10 to 25 percent. Most if not all of the additional sprint work should come at race pace, which isn't an all-out effort but rather the pace at which your priority event will be swum on race day. Those changes will add rest to the workout and fine-tune stroke efficiency at the most important speed and effort level.

In the early stages of tapering, the body begins to more fully recover from each workout before swimming the next because the muscle breakdown

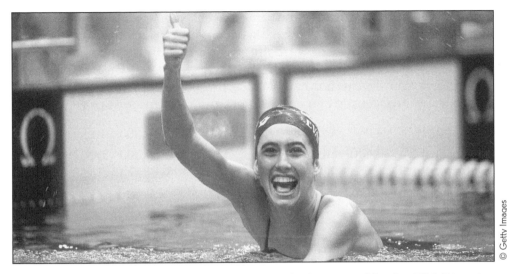

After tapering and shaving, I celebrated my victory in the 400-meter IM at the 1988 Olympics.

is decreasing with the decreased work load. As this catching-up process continues, you'll begin to feel like a new person. Because more and more of the minute muscle tears are repaired, you'll have more energy than you know what to do with during workouts. You'll start feeling really high in the water, you'll feel really good in every workout, and your speed will come more easily. If done correctly, the body becomes so fit and finely tuned that it becomes a ball of energy ready to burst off the starting blocks come race time. It's the ultimate fitness moment. The body is primed and ready to go fast, just in time for the race.

Although much is made of the tapering phase in talk and theories, this phase actually is an extremely short period of time. For example, I tapered for just 10 days for my first Olympics in 1988 after essentially swimming 18,000 yards (16,459 meters) a day for four years. The reduction in total distance is gradual and based on the distance and frequency of your regular workouts. The taper for athletes swimming four days a week and averaging 4,000 yards (3,657 meters) per workout should be about five workouts with about a 500-yard (12.5 percent) decrease in distance with each workout. The base attained at that distance and frequency would begin to decline if tapering lasted any longer or workouts were any shorter. The following is an example of a tapering program for such a swimmer.

| Day 12 | 4,000 yards | Day 6 | 2,500 yards |
|--------|-------------|-------|-------------|
| Day 11 | Off | Day 5 | 2,000 yards |
| Day 10 | 3,500 yards | Day 4 | Off |
| Day 9 | Off | Day 3 | 1,000 to 1,200 yards |
| Day 8 | 3,000 yards | Day 2 | Off |
| Day 7 | Off | Day 1 | Race day! |

Swimmers in the pool five or six times a week should reduce total distance swum by 10 percent of their normal workout every two days. For example, if you normally swim 4,000 yards per workout, you'll subtract 400 yards from your total every other day. Your final workout before the race should be about 25 percent of your normal distance, or 1,000 yards in this example. The following is an example of a tapering program for this type of swimmer.

| | | | |
|---|---|---|---|
| Day 15 | 4,000 yards | Day 7 | 2,000 yards |
| Day 14 | 3,600 yards | Day 6 | 2,000 yards |
| Day 13 | 3,600 yards | Day 5 | 1,600 yards |
| Day 12 | Off | Day 4 | Off |
| Day 11 | 3,200 yards | Day 3 | 1,000 to 1,200 yards |
| Day 10 | 2,800 yards | Day 2 | 1,000 to 1,200 yards |
| Day 9 | 2,400 yards | Day 1 | Race day! |
| Day 8 | Off | | |

The concept behind tapering is much easier to explain than to achieve. Because each swimmer is different from the next, and in fact might be different from one season to the next, the process is part science, part art. Hitting your taper can make all of the difference between winning a race and not making the finals, between achieving your goals or having to wait until the next season to try again.

There are two ways to miss a taper—being overtapered or undertapered—and the effect either way is fairly obvious during the race. Overtapered means you started your tapering workouts too far out from the race and, consequently, lost some of your conditioning. On race day, you start out fast because you're a bundle of speed and energy, but you hit the wall later in the race because your endurance level isn't what it needs to be. If you start to feel extremely fast a week or more before the race, bump up your base distance by 50 to 60 percent of what the tapering program calls for to keep your endurance level high. Overtapering happens to everyone, but distance swimmers are the most affected. Undertapered means you're overtrained. Either you didn't start tapering soon enough or you didn't adequately cut down on distance. The effect is a lack of the energy, zip, and freshness you want to feel on the starting blocks. The speed doesn't come easily, and neither does the distance.

Knowing when to start tapering, what distance to cut down to, and how to structure the workouts takes experience, a good read on your body, a fanatical dedication to recording every workout and race in your training log, and sometimes a little luck. When you nail it, you'll step onto the blocks through that small window of perfect fitness.

It's important to note that the tapering concept should be applied to all of your physical activity, not just your swimming. Any workouts you do other than swimming—weightlifting, yoga, Pilates, even sit-ups—should

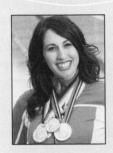

# Taper and Shave

The term "taper and shave" is common in swimming, especially in the world of competition. Like most swimmers, I really enjoyed the tapering phase. To taper meant a rare opportunity to rest and relax a bit during workouts and afterward, all in the name of training! But it also meant that race time was near, and race time was the payoff for all the hard work endured over the past several months or, in some cases, years.

The other half of the famous swimming phrase—shave—is no myth. Ever since the middle of the 20th century, swimmers have been shaving most or all of the hair off of their bodies in an effort to shave seconds off of their times in important meets. More than just a symbolic act, shaving makes a difference physiologically and psychologically.

Back before race suits covered much if not all of the body, the effect of shaving was more pronounced than it is today for swimmers wearing full-body suits. We would let the hair grow on our legs during the months of training. Then, the night before the meet, we'd have a big shaving party. My teammates and I would go to the store to buy shaving cream and then meet in one of our hotel rooms with our suits on. Everyone would crowd into the bathroom and take turns shaving in the tub. We'd shave our legs, our arms, and our backs. Thank goodness for swim caps or we would have been shaving our heads, too!

The next day in the pool, our sense of the water was extremely heightened because of the lack of hair on our bodies. The combination of tapering and shaving made us feel super fast in the water. Although both contributed to the overall effect of increased speed, it wasn't hard to recognize that tapering caused the more pronounced effect on us physically and shaving provided more of a mental edge. The result was the holy grail of swimming, when you stand up on the starting blocks feeling invincible, thinking, "Oh my gosh! I'm tapered! This is fantastic!"

also gradually decrease in length, time, reps, or intensity. Another important aspect of tapering is staying off your feet. Some swimmers spend their extra time shopping or running around with their friends, but the intent is to rest and save that energy for the race. Take advantage of the downtime by going to the movies or reading a book.

As you can see, tapering is a very small part of the formula that produces such dramatic results. Tapering only works if you've put in the hours, weeks, and months of hard work to build that fitness level and speed. The path through various stages and types of workouts to get to that point is just as important to success, though much less glamorous.

# Rest and Cross-Training

Also important to a swimmer's overall improvement from season to season is rest. Some people think their muscular strength and endurance gains take place during workouts, but in fact the opposite is true. During workouts, the muscles are broken down, and it's during the periods of rest between workouts that they repair themselves and get stronger. The tendency of some athletes to put in additional hours of training can be extremely counterproductive.

The body needs periods of rest each day. We physically can't work out 24-7. The body also needs periods of rest each week. Working out seven days a week is not smart. Even Olympians give their bodies a break one day a week. If you find yourself dragging through your days and your workouts, allow yourself an extra day off a week or sleep in one morning during the work week. Your workouts and disposition will benefit from it.

Likewise, a swimmer's yearly schedule should include periods of near-total rest and cross-training. The body cannot handle intense training year-round, just as the mind cannot concentrate for weeks on end without the breaks that evenings, weekends, or vacations allow. "Vacations" from focused physical activity are imperative not only to success and health but to the pure enjoyment of the activity. Early burnout is often the result of too grueling a schedule for too long a time.

For two to three weeks after each season ends, your time in the pool should be curtailed drastically, if not cut completely. Fill the time with physical activity that feels more like play than work: leisurely walks or bike rides, gardening, or participating on recreational sports teams. But only for two to three weeks—any longer than that and your fitness levels will begin to decline. After that short break, the intensity can be increased gradually for the next several weeks, but it's still best to limit your time in the water. Begin lifting weights again, go back to yoga and Pilates classes, and get most of your endurance work outside of the pool. Depending on what you like to do and where you live, the possibilities are numerous: walking, jogging, biking, cross-country skiing, hiking, climbing stairs, and using the elliptical machine are just a few possibilities. The rejuvenation of the body and mind helps you arrive at the start of the next base phase fresh and ready to work hard.

# appendix

# Converting Workouts for Metered Pools

The workouts in this book are designed for a 25-yard pool. Almost all intervals in the main sets of freestyle workouts are on a 1:00 per 50-yard base. If you are swimming in a 25- or 50-meter pool, as opposed to a 25-yard pool, you should alter the interval base in these workouts to account for the difference in length between yards and meters. Fifty yards equals 45.72 meters, or 91.4 percent of 50 yards. A good rule of thumb is to add five seconds per 50 meters when converting from yards to meters. Instead of a base of 1:00 per 50 yards, you would use a base of 1:05 per 50 meters. If you are swimming in a 50-meter pool, stop at the halfway mark when the workout calls for swimming 25 yards. Similarly, when swimming the 100 IM workouts in chapter 9, switch strokes at the halfway mark.

# references

Robergs, R.A., and R. Landwehr. 2002. The surprising history of the "HRmax = 220 – age" equation. *Journal of Exercise Physiology* 5 (2): 7. (http://faculty.css.edu/tboone2/asep/Robergs2.pdf)

Sleamaker, R., and R. Browning. 1996. *Serious training for endurance athletes*. 2nd ed. Champaign, IL: Human Kinetics.

# index

# about the author

**Janet Evans,** three-time Olympian and four-time individual Olympic gold medalist, is considered the greatest female distance swimmer of all time. By age 11, she was setting national age-group records, and in 1987 she set world records in the 400-, 800-, and 1,500-meter freestyle. At the 1988 Olympics, her first, she won gold medals in the 400- and 800-meter freestyle and the 400-meter individual medley. She captured gold again at the 1992 Olympics in the 800-meter freestyle and took silver in the 400-meter freestyle. After her 1988 performance, Evans continued to dominate the American and world distance scene. She became the first woman ever to win back-to-back Olympic and World Championship titles in any event, adding the 1991 and 1994 World titles to her Olympic golds in the 800-meter freestyle.

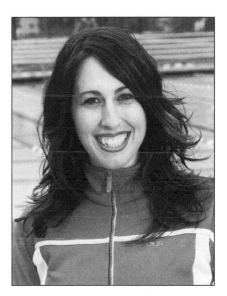

Evans was named the Female World Swimmer of the Year by *Swimming World* magazine in 1987, 1989, and 1990, and she won the Sullivan Award (top amateur athlete in the United States) in 1989. At the end of her career, she held 6 U.S. records, 3 world records, 5 Olympic medals (including 4 gold), and 45 U.S. national titles. She won the 400- and 800-meter free at the U.S. National Championships 12 times each, the most national titles in one event by any swimmer in the 100-year history of the event.

Evans' Olympic career ended in 1996, when she was honored with the prestigious task of passing the Olympic torch to Muhammad Ali, who lit the cauldron. She still holds world records in the 800- and 1,500-meter freestyle, both of which are the longest-standing records in the sport. Her record in the 400-meter freestyle held for 18 years until it was broken in May of 2006. Since her retirement, Evans has been a sought-after motivational speaker and corporate spokesperson for companies such as AT&T, Speedo, Campbell's, PowerBar, John Hancock, Cadillac, and Xerox. Evans also conducts youth swim clinics and hosts the Janet Evans Invitational Swim Meet, which is now in its 14th year.

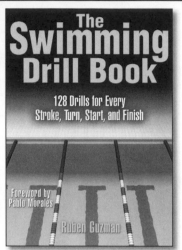
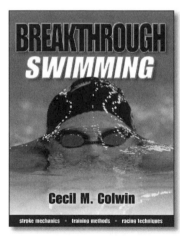